Navel Gazing

One Woman's Quest for a Size Normal

ANNE H. PUTNAM

FABER & FABER

First published in 2013
by Faber and Faber Limited
Bloomsbury House
74–77 Great Russell Street
London WC1B 3DA
This paperback edition published in 2014

Typeset by Faber and Faber
Printed and bound by CPI Group (UK) Ltd, Croydon, CR0 4YY

A CIP record for this book
is available from the British Library

978-0-571-28445-0

2 4 6 8 10 9 7 5 3 1

To you, for reading this. Thank you.

Author's Note

This book is a work of non-fiction, but assembling it has sometimes necessitated the use of creative license: some names have been changed, and some scenes or conversations are examples of typical moments from my life, rather than word-for-word retellings. While the story and its core events are all true, this book was written from a single perspective – mine – and my memory is far from infallible.

My gastric bypass operation was performed over a decade ago, at the beginning of the weight loss surgery revolution we seem to be experiencing now. Please bear in mind that my memories of my own surgery may not reflect the way things are done now – if gastric bypass is something that interests you, I beg you to do your research and speak with the appropriate medical professionals. This is just one person's story, and should not be taken as a medical reference, nor should it be seen as either an endorsement or a denunciation of weight loss surgery as a whole.

Diagram of gastric bypass surgery

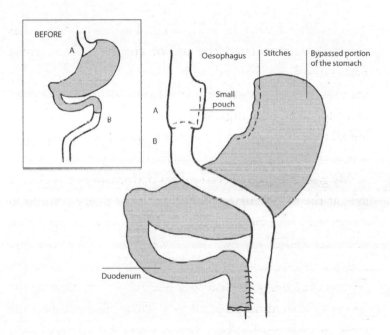

Conversion charts

Weight conversions

100 lb	7 stone 2 lb	45.4 kg
200 lb	14 stone 4 lb	90.7 kg
250 lb	17 stone 12 lb	113.4 kg
260 lb	18 stone 8 lb	117.9 kg
290 lb	20 stone 10 lb	131.5 kg

Dress size conversions

US	UK
8	12
10	14
12	16
14	18
16	20
18	22
20	24

Prologue

San Francisco, California, April 2001

Sixteen years old

Giggles and shouts echo off the tile walls around me. I shut my eyes for a second and try to imagine myself somewhere else, but the damp smell of chlorine refuses to let my mind wander. I open my eyes again and stare at the door of the bathroom stall in which I've barricaded myself. I look down at the one-piece swimsuit in my hands; I've twisted and wrung it until it's barely recognisable. My knuckles are white, and my hands are trembling a little.

'Anne!' My friend Tessa is shouting from the locker room. 'Anne, are you almost ready? We have to be in there!'

I take a shaky breath and shout back, 'Yeah, I'll be out in a sec, just tell the coach I'm being slow!'

I hear the door swing open and bang against the lockers, and someone giggles, 'Whoops!' and then it's quiet.

I sigh, stand up off the toilet seat, and pick my right leg up to put it through the hole in my suit. The elastic around the opening starts to stretch as I pull it past my knee, and I leave it for a minute while I put my left leg through, losing my balance and slamming my hand against the wall in the process. When I've got the suit about halfway up my thighs, I pause and stand up straight, giving myself a second to breathe. The last thing I want is to come out into the pool looking all sweaty and red-faced from the exertion of encasing myself in spandex.

I keep my eyes trained on the hook on the back of the door, where my yellow-and-white-striped towel is hanging. My last line of defence. My gaze traces the terry loops, runs up the borders and down the stripy centre – anything to keep from looking at my body, which I can feel spilling out of my swimsuit already.

I bend down and grab the straps of my suit. I pull hard, trying to make the process as quick as possible; the suit takes a second to move, but once it starts it slithers evenly up my body like a slow, persistent tidal wave, pushing mounds and rolls of fat out of its way until it extends to its full length. I tug the top over my breasts, tuck them in and pull the straps over my shoulders, then I focus on arranging my belly inside the slippery casing of the suit. Finally, I pull the leg holes up and out from my body, relieving myself of a wedgie and re-arranging the rolling hills of hip that have been trapped in awkward positions. When I let the material snap back into place, it digs into my flesh, causing mounds of thigh to escape from the taut smoothness of my elastic-corseted torso.

I grab the towel off the hook and wrap it around myself, tucking it in under my armpits. I take another deep breath, smooth my hair behind my ears, and unlock the door. I have to stand over the toilet so the door can open all the way, and then I sidle out into the locker room. I look at the clock – I'm already five minutes late. Coach is probably going to shout at me, but with any luck I can get into the water while my classmates have their faces submerged, swimming laps. I turn toward the exit, steeling myself for the moment when I have to remove my towel, but I'm caught by my own reflection.

My face is red, my hair is frizzing, and my upper lip is a little sweaty from the wrestling match with my one-piece. Below the neck, I'm just a mound of yellow and white. I hold my breath and slowly open the towel. Tears prick my eyes as I force myself to look at my body. It's massive. My breasts are too small for my frame, and look fat rather than full; my hips are rolling out of the suit like uncooked dough squishing out of a too-small bowl; my wide stomach is stretching the shiny black fabric to the max, and my belly button is outlined like a doughnut; beneath the suit, my thighs are white and red and dimpled, the skin pressed together down to the knees, where my legs splay out, making a triangle of space that ends at my pudgy feet, six inches apart.

I'm horrified by myself, and paralysed. I stand there, staring at this hideous girl who's wearing my face, my hands touching the slick material on her belly, until I hear the door open.

In a flash, I'm covered in the towel again. I wipe my eyes and walk into the locker room. Coach is standing in the doorway, looking harassed, but she stops when she sees my red eyes.

'Come on, Anne,' she says in a gentler voice than I've ever heard from her, 'let's go. Your friends are waiting for you.'

I nod, and follow her out into the open.

I

BEFORE

I

Manhattan Beach, California, June 1993

The inner thighs of my bike shorts swish past each other and my jelly sandals – purple of course, like everything else I'm allowed to choose – squeak a little, my feet slipping around in them as I trot down the hill, trying to keep up with Andrew. The pavement is already hot, burning the soles of my feet even through my shoes, and the Southern California sun is beating sparkles into the ocean that stretches out in front of us. I squint against the glare and try not to think about all the girls down on the beach in their bikinis, flirting and laughing and not wearing huge T-shirts over their swimsuits to protect them from sunburn and shame.

I've always loved living in Manhattan Beach. Our house is three blocks from the water, and my best friend lives a couple of streets over, just through the top of Sand Dune Park. We spend our weekends on the beach, making sand castles and trying to ignore Andrew, and pretending we don't think his best friend, Scott, is super-hot. I love where I live. But lately, since I started the third grade and turned

3

eight, things have started to feel ... different. I have these new classmates – they're twins, and everyone remembers which one is which because one is chubby, like me. I never realised or cared before that all my friends are skinnier than I am, but now the thought of sitting on the beach with them in nothing but our swimsuits makes me feel squirmy.

Andrew crosses the street without looking, and I swallow a cry of protest and launch myself after him. His long legs glide easily over the pavement – he got my mom's body type, slim and leggy, while I'm stuck with my dad's long torso and heavy frame, and have to move my legs twice as fast as he does to keep pace. He barely looks at me as I catch up; he's probably embarrassed to be seen with his fat little sister, but he needs a partner in crime. We both do.

When we reach Manhattan Avenue and turn left, the sign comes into view: Moon's Market. Right next door to the pizza place with the surfer on the logo, which is next door to the deli where our older sister, Catie, sometimes works when she comes home from college in the summers. As we pass the deli, I start planning how I'm going to spend my allowance; we each have a ten-dollar bill, which goes pretty far at Moon's.

We duck into the heavy cool of the store and pause, relishing the shade, letting our eyes adjust after the brightness outside. I hover in front of the candy stand, running my tongue over the inside of my mouth to try to figure out what kind of candy I'm craving. Fruity? Chocolatey? Crunchy? Sour? I reach for the bright yellow pack of Starburst, then pull my hand back – *too crinkly, Mom might hear*. I choose

4

the milder, slightly waxy Mambas instead. Starburst Lite. Less flavour, less packaging, just as much sugar and satisfying chew. *Still fat-free, at least.*

I can feel Mr Moon watching me. I wonder if he's thinking we might steal something or if he just thinks I'm too fat to be eating all this candy. I try to ignore him, focusing as hard as I can on the chocolate-toffee Heath bar in my left hand, but the hot, prickly blush invades my face anyway. I wish he would do something, move around, but he always stays behind the counter, watching.

Now I have two candy choices in my collection, one fruity and one chocolate, but I want more. Who knows when I'll get the chance to come back? Mom doesn't leave us alone often, and never for long. I scan the racks, thinking not only of flavour but of longevity too; I can't very well hide a pint of Cookies 'n' Cream ice cream under my bed or in my Barbie shoebox. I grab M&Ms, plain, and red liquorice Twizzlers, then pull back again for one last look. I hear the door to the refrigerated case close and turn to see Andrew standing over my shoulder. He reaches over me to grab a KitKat bar – he already has a big bottle of Pepsi under his arm.

'That's it?' I'm desperate for him to buy more, to even us out and make me less a glutton than a deprived child of a health nut. He looks at the pile of brightly coloured wrappers in my arms, and the burn spreads across my cheeks again. Andrew sees, and looks away.

'Let's just pay and get out of here. Mom'll be home soon.'

I lay my plunder on the counter and unfurl the bill I've

been clutching in my palm; it's hot and limp, and a little damp. Mr Moon takes it slowly, but instead of getting my change he just stares at me. I shift my weight to my other foot and look at the counter. My purple feet. The cold, blue-grey cement floor.

'Does your mother know you're here?' His voice is deeper than I expected, more masculine than his slight, bent frame would suggest. His eyes are narrowed at me; I feel like I've been busted for shoplifting, or worse, like I've been caught buying candy behind my mother's back. Which, of course, I have been.

'Of course she does.' Andrew speaks up with a voice steadier than my whole body. 'Don't you think our parents would *find out* if we were sneaking out of the house all the time?'

I'm not sure his bluff has worked, but Mr Moon pushes a button on the register and hands me my change without another word, and we flee into the sun's harsh glare.

'Jeez, that was close! Do you think he'll tell on us?' I'm panting – the way back home is all uphill. I try to swallow my heavy breaths and ignore the stinging in my calves.

Andrew barely looks at me, just shrugs and grunts. His stride is almost double the length of mine, and he takes the hill easily.

'Whatever. That old dude probably doesn't even know who Mom is. When was the last time you saw her go into Moon's? Or even the pizza place?'

I exhale in relief. He's right. Mom only shops at the grocery store, and she would never go into the pizza place. Only

Dad takes us there, although Mom might order a delivery from them on special occasions.

'Yeah, OK.'

We walk in silence, the only sounds my huffing and puffing and the squeak of my rubber shoes on the asphalt. Andrew drinks half his Pepsi on the way home, but I've got all my candy stuffed carefully into my waistband under my big T-shirt. I never eat it until I can really savour it, alone in my room.

By the time we reach our street, I'm trailing a good twenty feet behind Andrew, and he's getting fed up. When he gets to our front gate he stops and turns, placing his fists on his hips with exasperation.

'Come *on*. Mom's gonna get home soon and want to know where we were!'

I glare at him, but I don't quite have the breath to say anything in response without embarrassing myself further.

'Come on, Annie,' Andrew puts his hands on his thighs like he's calling a dog, 'snap, crackle, pop, burn that fat!'

I feel like I've been slapped. My face, already hot from the weather and the hill, burns until it stings, and tears gather at the corners of my eyes. I will them to go away – nothing entices further torture like the sight of tears.

As I reach my brother, I glance up at him, just to show him I'm not afraid, and to hiss 'Asshole' in his direction. The bad word feels less powerful than I thought it would, but for a second I think Andrew might feel kind of bad for saying what he did. Then he spots the tears, and the possibility of having to show real remorse stops his pity cold.

'Oh, what, now you're gonna *cry*?'

'No!'

Yes.

Andrew scoffs at my tears and pushes through the front door. I give myself a minute to calm down, kick at the gate as if it might be on his side, and then follow him in.

The house is cool, quiet. I know it won't be empty for long, so I head straight to my room to stash my candy. The chocolates have become a bit squidgy from being so close to my warm belly, but they'll firm up eventually. I hide the treats in different parts of my room, so that if one is found the others will be safe, and nobody will ever figure out just how much I hoard at one time. I wedge the Twizzlers inside one of my shoes, the white patent Mary Janes that are too stiff to wear. The Heath bar is flat, so it fits in between the pages of *Teen Bop*, in my nightstand. The M&Ms I stuff into my underwear drawer, careful to cover them with plenty of Disney Princess panties.

The Mambas, though, I hang onto for a minute. I really want to eat one or two before my mom comes home and smells the artificial fruit flavours on my breath. I open the package and take out two of the raspberry ones, tiny rectangles wrapped individually with a waxy paper. I tuck the rest of the Mambas in between the mattress and the headboard, and sit down on my bed to slowly unwrap the first of the two allotted candies.

I pop the Mamba in my mouth and fold up the wrapper into smaller and smaller squares, until it's barely visible. The candy on my tongue is soft, and warm from the trip. It doesn't have much flavour besides sweet, with a hint of berriness. I hold it there in my mouth without chewing for a minute, savouring the taste of refined sugar and the texture of taffy, then I let myself bite it. Once. Twice. And then I swallow. It's all over too fast, and I'm glad I've grabbed another. The second piece is gone almost as quickly as the first, although this time I pause to let the partially chewed candy squish between my two front teeth, where there's a big gap that gets bigger every year. The sound is hideous, but it feels delicious.

Just as I've swallowed the candy, and am allowing myself to consider grabbing another, I hear the front door open and my mom calls out a greeting. I leap off the bed, call back, and rush to the bathroom to scrub the scent of sugar off my teeth and tongue.

Andrew and I went on these candy-seeking excursions as often as we could – whenever my mother left us alone in the house for more than ten minutes or we could think of an excuse to 'go on a walk' together. They were some of the few occasions where we willingly spent time together, and they were the roots of a lasting bond; my brother and I were united in our rebellion against our mother's healthy kitchen.

We were partners in candy-sneaking crime, and we kept each other's secrets – I didn't tattle when he hid his asparagus in the African violet on the dining table, and he never snitched about the stash of sweets in my bedroom. We moaned in tandem after visits to friends' houses, where Girl Scout cookies and bags of potato chips sat unguarded in low cupboards, accessible to all. We told anyone who would listen about our sugar-free prison – wildly exaggerated tales of carob-chip 'cookies' and fruit for 'dessert'.

But there was something that separated us in our fight for fructose: I was fat, and Andrew wasn't. To be fair, I wasn't really tormented for it; my family was much more in-to ridicule and torture of each other's intellectual failings. I can count on one hand the number of cruel comments my brother ever made about my weight, which is exactly why, unfortunately for him, I remember every instance as sharply as if he'd just said it an hour ago. But still, my weight prob-lem was never far from anyone's mind; it was always there under the blubbery surface. I was the elephant in the living room.

Andrew was naturally thin; he had my mother's long legs and straight body. But he also shared my mother's active life-style: he sought out games of pickup basketball, rollerbladed for fun, and was satisfied with one small bar of chocolate. I, on the other hand, would much rather read a book than run a lap, and would stop at one piece of candy only if that was the limit of the offer. We were both normal kids, with nor-mal childish sweet teeth, held hostage by the Wicked Witch of the Watercress, like a reverse Hansel and Gretel. But we were also very different from each other, and it showed, not just on our bodies but also in the way we were treated.

For all our dramatic complaints, sugar wasn't completely banned in our house. There were birthday cakes, and Christ-mas stockings stuffed with malt balls, and once I even had a Valentine's Day cookie-decorating party, when the house was strewn with heart-shaped sugar cookies dripping with pink royal icing. But the few non-holiday treats we got, the flukes, those were all down to Andrew.

Intentionally or not, our parents treated us differently. At a restaurant, when the waitress asked if we wanted to see the dessert menu, I'd hold my breath and telepathically beg Andrew to say yes before my mom could say no. I rarely said anything, for fear of the awkward silence while my parents tried to figure out how to nix the idea without hurting my feelings and starting a sulk. The same was true of grocery shopping – I'd linger over the Fruit Roll-Ups or snack packs, hoping Andrew might catch my drift and decide he wanted them too.

He didn't always get what he wanted – far from it – but he didn't get a loaded response, either. When Andrew asked for something, the response was usually 'Don't be ridiculous,' or sometimes 'OK, just this once, but only if you stop hiding your green beans in the houseplants and start eating them!' But it was never an uncomfortable pause and a guiltily stuttered reminder of 'what the doctor said about your weight being a bit high ...' To me, Andrew seemed so bold – I wouldn't *dare* ask for Cookie Crisp instead of Cheerios just because my friend got Rice Krispies Treats cereal – but to him it was just a request, and sometimes a negotiation, and the worst our parents could do was say no.

But if Andrew had an easier time of it with my mom, at least I had my dad – when he was home from his never-ending business trips. See, I wasn't the only portly one in the family; my dad was also thickening more around the middle every year. And just like she watched what went into her own mouth and her kids' mouths, my mom tried to monitor my dad's habits as well. But Dad was a grown-up, even if he didn't act like one; he had a car, and money, and the same rebellious sweet tooth we kids had. It was a dangerous and fun combination.

Dad and I were two peas in a plus-sized pod. Whereas my mom and brother were generally quiet, shy, and slender, Dad and I were loud, bombastic, and rotund. It was the family divide: the WASPy Wamplers, my mother's matriarchal family, and the Pudgy Putnams, my dad's knock-kneed, pear-shaped clan. I knew exactly where I fit in. So it was no surprise that I was Dad's first choice for his 'adventures', as he called them. Later, we started calling it FaDaBoTi: Father–Daughter Bonding Time. And what is more bonding than food?

For us, food was at the clogged heart of FaDaBoTi. Dad would come home from a business trip on a Thursday, spend about twenty-four hours playing with us and chatting with my mom and talking about how good it was to be home, and then by Friday afternoon he'd have itchy feet again. This was perfect timing for the rest of the family: Andrew and I would be running around the house, getting in my mom's way, fighting and shouting at each other and yelling for parental intervention – 'Moooooooooom, Andrew's touching me when I told him not to *touch me*!' – and my dad would open the front door, jingle the car keys, and wait for the thundering of our feet. We would pile into the car, pausing to fight over who got the front seat, and head off to a movie or an illicit lunch of burgers and root-beer floats.

The big stuff – the movies; the winding drives through surrounding neighbourhoods; the odd trip to Disneyland – always included both kids. But as Andrew got older and spent more of his weekend with friends, the trips out of the house just for food lost his interest. Not mine, though. I was always up for a meal out with my dad; it meant precious alone time with a father who was away a lot, and it also meant a break from the healthy sandwich-and-fruit lunches of home.

Even Dad policed my eating habits sometimes, although I suspected he was doing it either to snag some of my food or to take his focus off his own perpetual diet (he'd been a runner when he met my mom, and only started putting on serious amounts of weight when he started his own company and began working such ridiculous hours that he barely had time to sleep, let alone run ten miles or eat a normal meal). He would reach across the table for a handful of my fries, saying, 'Here, let me save you from yourself,' or he'd catch me eyeing the dessert menu and yank it roughly from my hands, saying, 'Come on now, you don't want dessert.' But most of the time it felt like the two of us against the world (or my mother's watchful eye), and we padded our fortress with Philly cheese steaks and Häagen-Dazs and liquorice-rope Red Vines. We would go out and be free; Dad could drive like a crazy person and my mom wasn't there to white-knuckle the dashboard, and I could order a milkshake or curly fries without the fear of her furrowed brow. We were like two cons escaped from a prison of healthy, balanced meals and sensible life choices.

Of course, the minute we got home, he would flip to the other side again: parents together as one, the Parental Unit. But I clung to the feeling of it being our little secret, the invisible wink he would give me while telling my mom we'd just grabbed a quick bite, omitting the name of the restaurant or what we'd ordered. I doubt my mother was unaware of our doings – she wasn't unaware of much – but I suspect she let it go on because she was tired of policing. It's exhausting, always being the strict one, especially when you have to watch out for your kids *and* your husband.

So the FaDaBoTi went on, and I revelled in it, especially because outside the family unit I was becoming more and more uncomfortable about food. I was aware that I was getting fatter every year; my paediatrician had been telling me to lose weight since I could remember, and there were even a few more serious attempts made. Sweets and fatty foods had always been kept for special occasions, but I was starting to get the message that they really should be avoided altogether. Exercise wasn't about fun any more, my parents trying to get me into rollerblading because it was the next big thing; now it was about burning calories and 'getting fit'. My mother even took me with her to a Weight Watchers meeting once – she was constantly worried about losing or maintaining her weight, although to me she looked very slim and she had always been healthy by any standards – but I just zoned out and tried not to look as bored as I felt. All I got out of that hour was a vivid image of a pair of fat hands with acrylic, fire-engine-red fingernails, gesticulating wildly while a woman's voice droned on about spaghetti and meatballs.

But even as I resisted my mother's attempts to curb my weight gain, the knowledge that there was something wrong with my body, and that it was connected with food, seeped in. I began to feel self-conscious eating candy in front of my friends; I would practically force them to eat it with me, as if by sharing the sweets they also shared the burden of guilt. I started refusing offers of cookies at other people's houses, and taking smaller pieces of cake at birthday parties, only to overindulge when given the chance to do so in private. I discovered how it felt to resist my own greed, the satisfaction that came with denying myself something I was desperate to have, the respect people gave me for 'being good'.

But it wasn't just my relationship with food that was changing – I was also beginning to be more aware of my body as an asset or drawback to my overall appeal. Instead of looking at my best friend's bathing suit when we played on the beach, I noticed her long legs and firm belly. I wondered whether the reason my mother made me wear one-piece swimsuits was less because she thought bikinis on little girls were 'inappropriate' and more because bikinis on chubby girls were unappealing. And at ten years old, on a class field trip to a diving school, when the instructor was getting wet suits for us and asked if anyone weighed over a hundred pounds (I weighed 105), I found out that the number on the scale meant more than just a lecture from the doctor at my yearly physical. It meant I was *abnormal* in some way, and could even keep me from enjoying the same activities as my friends. So I learned to hide it; when I told my friends that day that I weighed five pounds too much they tried to convince me to tell the instructor, but I couldn't. I was paralysed by fear of humiliation, and shame. I never talked about my weight in a casual way again.

In those days, I was still just *chubby*: rounded belly, thick thighs. I was a fledgling fat, but I had started to notice the ways my body made me different from everyone else, and I didn't like it. I started to pray at night, to a God I wasn't even sure I believed in, reading the words off an old crocheted square that hung in a frame on my bedroom wall:

> Now I lay me down to sleep
> I pray thee Lord my soul to keep.
> If I should die before I wake
> I pray thee Lord my soul to take.

After the rhyme, I would add my own touch: 'Dear Lord, please protect me and everyone I love, especially my family. Please help me be healthy and safe, and lose weight. Thank you, I love you, amen.'

I said that prayer every night, lying on my back, staring up at the ceiling and willing myself to imagine a kindly old man just beyond, listening. I even prayed at sleepovers, silently chanting the words in my head with my eyes scrunched shut, hoping God could hear thoughts.

I still had faith then. I thought everything could be better if I just got thin: my family would relax around me; I wouldn't have to dread my yearly checkups with my doctor;

I could wear a swimsuit on the beach without a big T-shirt over it. Best of all, I could eat whatever I wanted in front of people, because I'd be normal. I thought maybe people were right when they said it was just 'baby fat', maybe I'd grow out of it as I got older. Maybe as I got taller, and grew into my teen years, I would stretch up instead of out, and the fat would turn into lean, long muscle.

I held onto hope that when I went through puberty, my body would change for the better: I would get taller like my brother, my legs would lengthen like my mother's, and I would grow beautiful, pert breasts like the girls I saw on the beach every weekend. As it happened, though, puberty would only worsen the problem: I would keep gaining weight; the attempts at healthy eating and activity would become ever more desperate diets and fads; and, worst of all, as I began to enter into the world of women I would place even more importance on how I looked. And so would everyone else.

2

San Francisco, fall 1999

'Ooooooh! This one is *pretty*. You should try it on!' Andrea pulls a skirt from the overstuffed sales rack and thrusts it in my direction. Chiffon waves undulate my way and I catch glimpses of a graphic print – apples, maybe, or some sort of beetle? I bite my lip as I reach for it. *Beetles. Oh God, and tiny dragonflies too.* It's the prettiest piece of clothing I've seen all day, a perfect clash of floaty, romantic fabric and a cheeky, modern print, exactly my kind of thing. Since we moved to San Francisco four years ago, my interest in bike shorts and baggy T-shirts has waned, in favour of more feminine, stylish clothes, the kind I'm terrified will make me look like a potato in a dress.

When Andrea called this morning and asked if I wanted to go shopping with her, I figured it would be a day of wandering around, following her through stores and pretending I didn't like any of the clothes, giving her advice on outfits while I scanned the earrings and necklaces for something that I could buy. I didn't mind; I'd rather hang out with my friends in their world than invite them into mine. But

I didn't plan on her expecting me to participate. *Surely she knows I won't fit in anything here?* We haven't been friends for that long – about a year, since both our best friends ditched us for each other when we were thirteen – but I really like her. She's smart, and kind, and has parents who collect weird art with naked people in it, just like the embarrassing paintings that hang all over my house. She's one of the few people I feel truly comfortable around, partly because she's not all obsessed with losing five pounds and getting a boyfriend like most of the other girls at our middle school. We still haven't talked openly about my weight problem. I don't usually feel like discussing it, but maybe I should have; then maybe she wouldn't have such normal expectations of me.

I let out an exasperated puff of air and check the tag on the skirt she's holding out: XL. But then, that's an XL in Anthropologie, a gorgeous, expensive boutique full of beautiful, girly dresses and chic trousers, where even slim, athletic Andrea sometimes has to wear a Large. *But, oh, it's sooo pretty.* I run my thumb over the silky material, stroking a ladybug as I try to decide whether it's worth the potential humiliation. Whether I can even face the fitting-room attendant, who will probably take one look at my big, burgeoning hips and pink, pimply face and laugh me out of the store. Or, worse, she won't say anything, and her face will just scrunch up with anxiety at the imagined destruction of zippers and buttons.

'Anne?' Andrea has moved on and is now holding up a tangerine sweater, asking my opinion.

'What? Oh, yeah, really cute. That colour is gorgeous.'

'It's sooooo soft.' She rubs the cashmere against her cheek, then looks at the price tag. Her face falls, and she goes to put the sweater back where she got it.

I look down at the skirt again, and shake my head. *No. No way that would fit me.* I sigh, shove the hanger back onto the rack, and pick my way through the discarded cardigans and singleton shoes to Andrea, who's now contemplating a pair of pinstriped pants. She's already holding about seven hundred items in her arms. I wonder what it's like to be so unafraid. To try things on, just like that. To be a size medium. A size *normal*.

Andrea turns and sees that my hands are empty. She frowns.

'*What?* Where's that skirt? It would be so cute on you!'

I try not to blush as I shake my head. It's a losing battle.

'Oh, it wouldn't have fit me anyway. And besides, I only have forty dollars left from my allowance, and you know how Anthro is – that skirt probably costs like seventy bucks, even if it is on sale.'

I will her to accept the excuse and drop the issue, but instead she makes a scoffing noise and marches back to the skirts rack. It takes her a minute to find it again, but when she does, she pulls it triumphantly from the wreckage and reads the tag.

'See? XL, and it's only twenty-five bucks! You have to try it on. I mean, when was the last time you saw anything at Anthro that was this cheap? And besides, it's got *snails* on it! How *you* is that?'

I look at the skirt again. *Well, it is a circle skirt, so really the only part that would have to fit is the waist . . .* I reach for it, take it off the hanger, and hold the waistband up to my midsection. It looks like it might actually go all the way around.

'God, you have such a tiny waist.' Andrea looks at me almost enviously and I stare back like she's lost her mind. But she's serious – her body is pretty straight besides her round butt, while I'm all 'curves'. *If rolls count as curves.*

'Yeah, maybe compared to the rest of my massive-ass self!' I try to sound like I'm joking, but I push the skirt away from my body and cross my arms over my chest. *Like that'll hide anything.* 'Fine, whatever. I'll try it on if that'll make you happy. But when it doesn't fit and I'm sitting on the kerb crying into a pint of Häagen-Dazs and ruining my diet, it'll be your fault.' *Yeah, right, as if I'd give the world the satisfaction of seeing me cry into a tub of ice cream like their exact wet dream of a fat stereotype.*

Andrea pauses, and for a terrible moment I'm afraid she's going to try to talk to me about my body and my constant, ever-changing diet and my obvious self-loathing, which she's tried to do before because in her house everything is a grown-up conversation about social pressures and personal goals and strengths – I always find some way to change the subject, usually with a self-deprecating comment and a question about her latest healthy baking experiment. But this time she just rolls her eyes at me and heads for the dressing rooms. I breathe out the panic and follow, lingering to fondle soft angora sweaters and test lightly scented lotions.

When I finally get there, Andrea is already set up in a room. I call her name to find her.

'Yeah, over here!' A hand appears over the door at the end of the row. I flash a quick smile at the attendant, gesturing to my one item and my friend down the hall, and she nods warily and leads me to the room next to Andrea's. *Well, that's half the battle.*

The door clicks shut behind me and I'm alone in the dressing room, just me, a small wooden stool, some hooks on the wall, and the skirt. Oh, and a big, full-length mirror. I try not to look at it, but out of the corner of my eye, a monstrous figure comes into view, round and awkward, lumbering and uncomfortable. I turn to the wall, away from my reflection, and focus on the skirt.

The zipper comes down fairly easily, and I manage to get it over my head and shoulders OK. It's sitting on my hips now, skimming over my belly, and I chance a glance at the mirror to see how it might, theoretically, look if I can zip it up. I'm surprised by what I see; I look almost *girly*, with a defined waist and curvy hips. Without a normal person next to me for comparison, I can almost convince myself that I'm curvaceous, Rubenesque, and maybe even attractive in some parallel universe where waifish creatures like Gwyneth Paltrow and Claire Danes are snubbed in favour of chubbos like me.

I spin, and catch sight of the zipper, still undone. *Crap. Almost forgot about that part.* I close my eyes and take a deep breath, which I hold in my lungs until my heart pounds in my ears. When I finally breathe out I'm a little dizzy, which helps, because I can't really see my reflection very well. I suck my breath in again, pulling my stomach in with it, as far as it'll go. I grab the little pink tab on the zipper and tug. It slides easily up about halfway, then stops. I breathe out and examine it closely – it's just caught on the material. I free the silk and try again. It's slow going, but I get the zipper all the way up.

By the time I'm finished, my face is red and beginning to sweat, and my head is swimming. The waistband of the skirt is tight – it hurts a little, but I allow myself to hope that it's not unflattering. *Anyway, maybe if this new no-carb diet works, it'll be a bit more comfortable in a week or so.* As I turn slowly to face myself, I utter a quick prayer under my breath. *Please, God, I know it's been a while, but if you're out there, just give me this one thing. If you just let me look pretty in this one thing, I promise to try harder to have faith in you, even when I'm not on an airplane or really upset about my life.* I face the mirror.

No such luck. My fat spills out over the waistband in the unflattering way of suburban moms who've given up trying. I don't look horribly disgusting, but I do look like I need to go up a size. And, whether or not random passersby would know it, there *is* no 'up a size' for me. I've maxed out normal sizes. *Well, that's it, I guess.*

I feel the tears spring to my eyes as I fumble to undo the hook-and-eye closure at the top of the zipper. My skin is starting to hurt now where the waistband has been cinching it, but I ignore the pain and carefully extricate myself from the beautiful skirt. I breathe deeply, willing myself to stop getting so upset, stop crying. *Stop it, now. It is what it is – maybe if you stick to this diet and lose another ten or fifteen pounds you can come back. It's just a skirt.* Despite my efforts to calm myself, a tear escapes from the inside corner of my eye and rolls down my nose, tickling the tip before dropping onto my lip. I reach up and wipe it away, catching the drip from the inside of my nostril at the same time. I pull my corduroys up and fumble in my purse for a tissue. I should feel determined, steel myself to stick to this latest diet and then come back and spend a month's allowance at Anthro, but instead I just feel defeated. *What's the point of all this no-bread, salads-for-dinner shit if I can't even lose enough weight to get into a circle skirt?*

'Anne?' Andrea calls from right outside my door. 'Are you going to show me? I need to know what you think of this dress.'

I take a shuddery breath and wipe my face with the inside of my T-shirt.

'Yeah, I'll be out as soon as I'm decent. The skirt didn't work, but it's fine. Hey, at least it zipped up!' I try to sound cheerful, but I can hear Andrea feeling sorry for me. *I want to die. If I died right here, would it really be so bad? I mean, I'd be surrounded by beautiful things . . .*

I push past the sick feeling in the pit of my stomach, paste a smile on my face and wrench the door open. Andrea looks stricken by my blotchy face and puffy eyes, but I pretend not to notice, and hope she'll do the same. I try to keep the tremble out of my voice as I gesture at her outfit.

'Ooooh, *cute*! You have to get that – it's so girly and pretty!'

Andrea smiles and does a little spin in the dark blue dress she's trying on. Her hands fly to the floaty hem and she pulls the material away from her, almost like she's about to curtsy. She looks like a grown-up. A young *lady*. I tie my sweatshirt around my waist and settle into the couch, next to the guys whose girlfriends are trying things on. I smile awkwardly at the man next to me, then turn back to Andrea.

'Well, get back in there.' I make an ushering motion with my hand. 'I want to see the rest!'

*

When my family moved from suburban Los Angeles to urban San Francisco, I was jolted out of my comfort zone in more ways than one. Suddenly, not only were all my friends four hundred miles away, my laidback beach-bum lifestyle replaced with buses and hills, and my grassy front lawn switched for a dank, mossy, brick garden, but my childhood wardrobe was also made obsolete in the space of a seven-hour drive north in a U-Haul. San Francisco ten-year-olds didn't wear bike shorts and big T-shirts. They didn't run around in little girls' dresses and pigtails. San Francisco ten-year-olds wore jeans, and short skirts, and miniature versions of what San Francisco twenty-year-olds wore. I needed a whole new closetful of outfits, and this was going to be easier said than done.

Luckily, I went to an all-girls middle school that required uniforms, and I could just about fit in those, but 'free dress days', when we were allowed (or forced, as I saw it) to come to school in our own clothes, quickly became a source of stress. On the first free dress day, I wore Mary Janes and tights, a corduroy skirt, and a scoop-necked sweater – the nicest outfit I owned, besides the usual velvet Christmas dresses. I walked into school, still a new enough student that I felt nervous every morning, only to find that everyone was wearing jeans and 'baby-tees'. The nascent friendships I'd begun were tested by my first lie: when the girls asked why I was so dressed up, I told them that I was going to the symphony with my parents after school, and I wouldn't have time to change. That lie led to other, splinter lies, which I had to keep up for the rest of the week, as people asked me how the performance was and whether I really liked the symphony or my parents made me go.

As soon as I could manage it, I tagged along with my mom and brother to the sports store where he liked to get his jeans. I discovered that men's jeans usually fit me – they came in bigger sizes and were roomier in the hips and thighs than women's jeans – and for the first couple of years that I lived in the Bay Area, my weekend wardrobe consisted mostly of men's jeans and corduroys and hooded sweatshirts. It was comfortable, but it wasn't the easiest jumping-off point for exploring the changes that were happening to my body; there's not much you can do with newly budding breasts if they're hidden under a hoodie.

And then, one day, there was no more uniform. At fourteen, I graduated from eighth grade. My friends and I scattered to different high schools across the city; I went to a small, co-educational private high school where the dress code was simply 'as cool as you can afford to look'. Not only did I find myself in a completely new environment, with completely new people, half of whom were boys, but I was also in sudden need of a real, seven-days-a-week wardrobe.

I was thrust into the world of personal style, and I had no idea what mine was. All I knew was that I'd better find a way to figure it out, or I risked being more than just That Fat Girl – I risked being That Frumpy Fatty. Inconveniently, the summer between middle school and high school was when my body gave up straining at the limits of 'heavy' and 'chubby' and finally oozed over into the dreaded category of 'obese'.

Not much had changed about my lifestyle since we'd moved to San Francisco. I was still eating healthily at home, and still sneaking sweets with my brother (and, increasingly, on my own) when I had the chance. The cashier at the corner store by our new house wasn't as scary as Mr Moon, so maybe I went a bit more often, and because I was older I had more freedom and was allowed to go out with friends unsupervised, which frequently meant unhealthy meals and snacks. I was always on one diet or another – calorie-counting, fat-free, sugar-free, low-carb, no red meat – but they never lasted very long. I would screw my courage to the sticking place and be extremely strict with myself, and I would usually lose a few pounds in the first week, but after that it would get harder and harder to lose weight, and a five- or six-pound loss wasn't noticeable enough to keep me motivated. Eventually, I would fall off the wagon and give up, sliding back into the sinking certainty that I would never lose enough weight, and therefore never be good enough, never get a boy to like me, never be normal. And once I accepted that fact, I would fall back into old patterns and desires, sneaking food and eating carbs, until the next hot new diet or weight-loss fad caught my eye and I did it all over again.

Every new diet or exercise tape felt like a chance at normalcy, and I greeted each attempt with excitement and hope. But as I lost too little, plateaued quickly, and gained it back plus more over and over again, the hope diminished. In its place came resentment of my situation, which I didn't understand – why was it so hard for me? Why did I gain weight so easily and have such a hard time losing it? Some nights at the dinner table, while I devoured whatever low-calorie meal I was eating that night, I would look over at my thin brother, picking at his food (likely the same as mine, but more of it maybe), and anger and frustration would wash over me. I wanted what he had: a normal body; natural social confidence; a relationship with food that was just about need or desire, rather than being fraught with the thoughts of calories and fat content and carbs-vs-protein that twisted wickedly in my head at all hours of the day. The more I obsessed over which foods were 'good' and which were 'bad', the less I wanted to think about it – there were times when I had an opportunity to eat something forbidden, like a candy bar or a cupcake brought to school for someone's birthday, and I would eat it even if I didn't really want it, as if to prove to the world and myself that food didn't control me. That was all I wanted: to not be controlled by food, either because

I wanted it or because I couldn't have it. Either of those lives – the food-obsessive or the diet-obsessive – sounded entirely miserable to me, and I wanted to make sure I didn't go down either path. And the only way to do that was to lose weight.

Despite my diet and exercise attempts, though, I'd only been getting heavier, and every year my uniform size went up – by eighth grade I was wearing the biggest skirt the uniform place carried, and my mom still had to move the buttons over to make it fit – but even though I knew I was fat, and knew I was failing myself every time I stopped a diet and didn't go on another one right away, I didn't really register the *steepness* of my downward slide. Nor did anybody else, I think. I didn't go for regular checkups any more, now that we'd left the family paediatrician behind in Manhattan Beach, so I didn't have a steady track of how much I weighed, and when I started rapidly approaching the two-hundred-pound mark I panicked and stopped weighing myself so often at home. And I suspect that my parents, like me, were trying to avoid the awkward subject of my changing body. Nonetheless, that summer before I started high school I discovered that while I'd been hiding in XXL uniform skirts with the buttons adjusted, my body had changed beyond the usual adjustments; in addition to growing breasts and hips and armpit hair, I'd also outgrown the sizing at normal stores.

The timing of my discovery was especially unfortunate as my closest middle-school friends – Andrea and two other girls, Courtney and Sophie – had gone off to different high schools, and we spent our weekends reconnecting the way most fourteen-year-old American girls do: at the mall. We had all spent the past few years hidden behind pleated navy skirts and white sailor tops, and now we were helping each other develop our personal styles: Sophie, the soccer star, went sporty, choosing jeans and tanks and the odd low-cut top; Andrea took the sporty-cute California girl-next-door route, *ooh*ing and *aah*ing over feminine necklines and sundresses, but rounding out her closet with plenty of fitted jeans and shorts and sporty tops; Courtney, the artist of the group, liked to buy her basics in classic colours and shapes at expensive (for us) shops like Banana Republic and Club Monaco, but then she'd spend a few hours at the vintage stores in the Haight and add on interesting little bits and bobs, hats, belts, and sometimes full dresses or old-man cardigans.

We were all filling out our wardrobes after years of uniformed education, but because I had filled out more than the others I was relegated to offering advice on clothing and pretending I was only interested in accessories. And I *was* interested in them; when you're too big to shop at the same clothing stores as everyone else, the little things take on a lot of importance. I was horrified at the massive body I'd realised had been germinating while I was in middle school, but I was still determined to enter high school with some semblance of personal style, and things like nail polish, jewellery, and hairstyle were the easiest tools for expressing myself and playing with my appearance. But a girl can't dress herself in accessories alone.

In those days, 'plus-size fashion' was less about trends and more about covering up a shameful, dumpy body; my choices were limited pretty much to matronly, shapeless, unflattering shift dresses and long skirts, or worse: the high-waisted, tapered-leg mom jean. Shudder. There were a few exceptions, two of which became my go-to shops: GFLA (Girlfriends LA) was an online teenybopper-plus store that stocked cute, youthful outfits in sizes 0 to 28, and Lane Bryant, which was targeted more toward adults but didn't neglect young heavyweights, was a stylish plus-size chain for women of all ages and – most importantly – shapes. Not every fat woman is an apple. Some of us are pears to our cores.

My closest Lane Bryant was a forty-minute drive across the Bay Bridge, so I didn't go often. My sainted mother, though, spent enough money there every time we did go to make it worth her while to sign up for one of those in-store credit cards. It took serious savings to make my mom sign up for anything, so it's easy to imagine how much shopping we were doing. It was worth it, though, because those two plus-sized options were responsible for my high-school survival. Well, those stores and my tenacity.

No matter how I felt inside, no matter how much I hated myself and believed that I was worthless, outwardly I refused to play the fat-girl wallflower role. If I couldn't explore my sense of self and femininity the same way the other girls could – by coming to school in short skirts and belly shirts and lounging on the beach in string bikinis – then I was determined to at least remind the world that I was female. I may not have been a 'woman' in the sexy, seductive way I wished, but I could at least be a girly girl from the boobs up and the 'cankles' down. My stomach may have been pulling at the buttons on my shirt, my thighs may have bulged beneath my skirt, but my toes were impeccably polished, my earrings were unusual and colourful, and my hair was a distracting shade of cherry red.

Oh, and my tits were usually pushed up to the limit. The most common neckline in my high-school wardrobe was *plunging*. My favourite shirt was a pea-green knitted cotton top with a deep scoop neck; I loved it because it didn't cling to my rolls, and it drew attention to the little bit of collarbone that stuck out when I clasped my hands and pulled them away from my body. I wore that shirt every chance I got for the first two years that I owned it, and then one day, when I was sitting on a low wall waiting for the bus, a young man with eyes too wide to denote sobriety came right up to me, bent down and stared pointedly at my chest. When I asked if he was looking at my necklace (an egg-sized amethyst pendant Courtney had given me for my fifteenth birthday), he looked up into my eyes and cheerfully shouted: 'No! I'm looking at your cleavage!' I never wore that shirt downtown again; once faced with a real reaction to my breasts, I was forced to recognise my discomfort with any sort of objectification. I wanted my breasts to distract from the rest of me, but I didn't want people *looking* at them. I wanted to feel feminine, but in trying to show my breasts as proof of my femininity, I ended up feeling more like a tasteless joke than a woman.

So I kept at it, relying less on my breasts and more on creating a shape out of my lumps and bumps. Despite my girth,

I worked very hard to find clothes that fit me correctly and flattered what few assets I had, and generally I succeeded. I was desperate to look like the girly girl I felt I was inside, which sometimes led to my unfortunate over-flaunting of my breasts, but every now and then I did manage to make myself look and feel womanly. For a fat girl, I received quite a few compliments on my clothing, and I appreciated them more than people knew. I practically licked classmates' faces if they told me they liked my dress or my top. But hand in hand with the gratitude went panic; I was terrified they'd ask where I got the item, and I would have to admit that I was too fat for the Gap and had to buy my dresses online or at a plus-size store. Or, more likely, I'd have to lie and say I couldn't remember, or somebody bought it for me and removed the tag. Or some other bullshit that I was sure people saw right through.

And that fear of being found out applied to more than just the label on my jeans. Built into the fat was a sense of the ridiculous; I was terrified that if I tried too hard to look alluring or womanly I would end up a laughing stock, a mockery of sexiness, like a fat bearded man in drag. The few times I did move outside my comfort zone, I was reminded of my limitations. Like the time I decided that long fingernails were pretty and delicate – so I grew mine out and my sister stared at my hands, horrified, and said they looked like 'claws on potatoes'. I told her she was just jealous because *her* hands looked like a *man's*; I pretended I didn't care what she thought, but I also cut my nails that night and never let them grow long again.

Not that my sister was one to talk. She wasn't exactly a paradigm of femininity, and neither was my mother. That's not to say that either of them was mannish (Catie's hands weren't even mannish, just calloused and scarred from her new floral design business), but they were both kind of tomboyish in a preppy, attractive way. My mom was usually in jeans and a nice button-down shirt, and my sister occasionally wore a dress but then she'd throw a hoodie over it and stuff her hands in the pockets. Plus, they both had very different body shapes from me: my mother was straight up and down, and my sister was a bit top-heavy, while I had wide hips, a narrower waist, and relatively small breasts for my size. I had to find my own way, and all along I had to shore up my confidence in my decisions, so that when one of them looked at something I was wearing and made a comment that betrayed her misunderstanding of how fashion worked on a body other than her own, I could brush it off and know that I'd made the right choice.

Their personalities were just as confusing as their fashion choices – if I wanted to learn how to own and flaunt my womanliness, I certainly wasn't going to get it from them. My mom was the only feminine role model who was around regularly when I was growing up, and she was the quiet, WASPy type, more concerned with intellect and proper behaviour than girliness or feminine wiles. As for Catie, by the time Andrew and I had fully formed personalities she was already away at college, and the sister we knew from her school breaks could be summed up in our nickname for her: 'the belch queen'. And then there was my dad – loud, opinionated, and cranky – and my brother – crude, funny, and goofy. Somehow I ended up a strange mix of them all: a brash joke-cracking frat boy who liked pretty dresses and girly accessories, and who was usually barefoot but always had perfectly painted toenails.

I was torn between two desires: to be feminine and to be safe. I wanted people to see me as a girl, but I knew that if I encouraged the world to acknowledge my femininity I would make myself extremely vulnerable to rejection, the really painful 'you're too fat to be the type of girl people *like* to see' kind of rejection. Physically, I wished to be viewed as a young woman, but I was afraid my size would make that impossible. And if my femininity wasn't physically accept-able because it was covered in a thick layer of blubber, then I didn't dare show the world my *emotional* girliness. I would have to act like a guy, to throw them off the scent of my vul-nerability. So that's what I did.

My blunt, crude humour served me well as a fat girl. It helped distract people from the fact that I was supposed to be feminine, and amused them to the point where they didn't really care if I had breasts or not. To the girls, who were my sole classmates in middle school, I was a confidante, a friend, someone who would listen to their boy problems without ever needing help with my own – and to the girls who weren't my friends, I was too brusque and sturdy to be a victim, so I was never really bullied, short of a comment or two behind my back. To the guys, once I moved up to high school and met some, I wasn't a woman at all; I was just a dude in a dress. I hid my feelings for boys by mocking them and punching them on the arm. I treated every guy I met like I would treat my brother: with scornful affection.

Underneath my one-of-the-guys facade, though, I wanted desperately to be a real girl. I wanted to kiss a boy at a party and go squealing back to my friends with a blush spreading across my cheeks. I wanted to go shopping and blow my whole allowance on some beautiful, body-hugging dress and high heels that hurt my feet even as they made me feel like a woman. I wanted more than anything to be feminine, but I was too afraid to even try, terrified the world would point and laugh at my failed (fat) efforts.

So I straddled the line, five painted toes in the lush grass of girlish giggles and secret crushes, and one bare, calloused foot in the swamp of deep guffaws and fart jokes. But I couldn't hold that position for long. Eventually I would have to choose, and that would mean risking everything.

3

Santa Cruz, California, June 2001

I first spot him when I'm about halfway back to the rental house. He's across the street, walking his Dalmatian off-leash. He's cute, in a very Santa Cruz kind of way: skater-y, kind of chubby, but it looks like hard fat. Dark hair. Short, but taller than I am by a little bit. He looks kind of like the lead singer of the Barenaked Ladies, but then it's hard to tell, since I'm doing my best not to look interested.

He's crossing to my side of the street. I can hear his footsteps, and the dog's tag jingling; my pulse starts rushing as they get closer, and I try to control my breathing. God forbid I should be panting when he comes up on me. I move my arms slightly to see if I'm sweating – it's hot today, and my inner thighs are sticking together under my knee-length skirt, which is riding up a bit over my round hips. I'd like to adjust it but the bag in my arms is too heavy and anyway it'd be too obvious.

The dog gets to me first, jogging, the leash tied up and held in its mouth. I smile as it passes me, but it barely looks my way. I try not to take it personally; my mom always says Dalmatians are dumb as rocks from all the inbreeding.

'Hey.'

I turn. The guy has caught up with me. The sidewalk is too narrow for him to walk easily alongside me (although of course I don't blame the sidewalk), so I'm forced to look back over my right shoulder to see him. He *is* cute. Instead of feeling validated by this confirmation, I'm anxious. *What does he want?*

'Oh, hi.' I smile awkwardly and then focus my eyes in front of me, hoping he'll just walk off. Hoping he won't.

'Sorry about Al,' he nods at the dog, which is up ahead of us, peeing on somebody's roses. 'He's kinda antisocial.'

I turn and smile again. My neck is starting to hurt. I shift the bag of groceries to the outside arm, in case he tries to look in. There are cookies and chips in there. Not for me, of course – I'll try to allow myself only one or two cookies, which I will faithfully record in my food diary and balance out with celery sticks and salad tomorrow – they're for the party later today, but he wouldn't know that. I clear my throat so I don't sound as froggy as I feel.

'It's OK. I'm allergic anyway, and I probably wouldn't have been able to resist petting him and then I would have gotten all sneezy.' *Oh my God, why are you such a dumbass? Sneezy? Where did that come from anyway?*

He laughs. I'm still confused as to what he could possibly want with me. I step off the sidewalk and onto the grass lining the edge of the cement, in case he's trying to pass me and just doesn't know how to say 'Excuse me'. The grass is long and dry, creeping up over my flip-flops to tickle my toes; we haven't gotten nearly enough rain this year.

'So, do you go to school around here?'

'Um, no, I go to school in San Francisco. My cousin lives down here so we're just having kind of a family get-together sort of thing . . .'

'Oh, OK, that's cool. So you're here with your parents?'

'Yeah. Unfortunately.' I wonder if I'm fooling him. It's too weird for a sixteen-year-old to actually *like* hanging out with her parents.

'That's nice. You probably don't get to see them much.'

I look at him sideways, my brows furrowed, my head cocked.

He tries again. 'So let me guess, you're a . . . senior?'

I'm pleased he thinks I look eighteen, but I shake my head. 'Junior.' I'll start my third year of high school in a few weeks; I've had all summer to get used to the idea, but somehow it still feels weird not to be an underclassman any more, and to know that Andrew won't be there when I get back to school – he leaves for college in a couple months.

'Oh, OK. And you said San Francisco, right? USF or someplace else?'

I don't understand at first, and then suddenly I do. *He thinks I'm in college!*

'Oh! No, um, I'm a junior in high school.' I laugh nervously and wait for him to get all squirrelly and run off at the thought of jailbait. I'm surprised at myself for believing my instinct that I'm actually being flirted with.

'Oh! Damn! I thought you were at *least*, like, twenty.' He

smiles, but he doesn't run; he stays in step with me. He's leaving plenty of room beside him on the pavement, but I'm afraid I won't fit so I'm still picking my way through the grass, keeping an eye out for dog shit.

'No . . . I'm sixteen.'

Still no running. I feel strangely emboldened, and I decide to ask *him* a question this time.

'So . . . how old are you?'

'Twenty-six.' He cringes. 'I know. Old as shit, right?'

Yes.

'Nah. My sister's older than you are. Well, half-sister.'

'Oh, so you have siblings?'

'Yeah, two. I'm the baby.' *What is this, a first date?*

'That's cool. I've got a little brother. Although I guess he's not so little any more.'

We're getting close to the rental house, and I start to worry. *What if he's a creepster and he just wants to see where we're staying so he can rob us or something? Why did I tell him we're not from here?*

I realise I'm probably overreacting, that I was probably right to think this guy was normal and cool in the first place, but the mere fact that he's flirting with me has me coming up with crazy scenarios in which he's using me for something. Normal, *cute* guys don't flirt with me. I don't want him to see where the house is though, just in case, so I pause a block before the street where I need to turn right.

'Um, I have to turn here, so . . .'

He looks disappointed.

'Oh, OK, well it was cool talking to you . . . ?'

'Anne.' *Oh, should have given him a fake name, but I can never think of one fast enough.*

'Anne. Nice talking to you. I'm Chris.'

'Nice to meet you.'

We stand there on the corner for another minute. I don't want to just walk away. Not only does that seem rude, but also this guy is cute! *But I don't know him at all. And he lives in Santa Cruz. And he's probably a creeper, anyway.*

I turn to leave and he puts a hand out, lightly touching my bare arm. I feel the hairs on my skin stand up.

'Hey, Anne. I'm going down to the beach?' He points toward the water and raises his eyebrows, waiting for my confirmation that I know where the beach is. 'My friend is working at this cafe down there, Curly's. I'll be there all afternoon, just hanging out. You should come chill if you're free later.'

I have no idea how to react. *Did he just ask me to hang out? Like, a date?* I try to control my cheeks, but they blush despite my best efforts.

'Um ... Yeah, maybe? I mean, I'd like to, it's just I don't know whether my family has plans for the rest of the day ...' A complete lie. No plans until the party, which isn't for hours.

'OK, cool. Well, I'll hope to see you there, anyway.' He smiles, and the skin at the corners of his eyes creases. *God, he's really cute.* 'Have a good time with your family.'

'Yeah, you too, with your friend.' I turn and walk off down the wrong street, hoping I can double back at the end of the block. Trying to breathe through all the possible scenarios running through my mind. Trying to keep one foot in front of the other despite my quivering knees and slightly blurred vision. *Oh my God oh my God oh my God. This has got to be a prank. He's made a bet with his friends to pick up the saddest chick he can find and bring her to the bakery for a cupcake with a free side of humiliation. Yeah, this is definitely one of those bad teen-movie moments.*

I resist the urge to glance back down the street as I round the corner, telling myself he's already headed toward the beach. Hoping he's not standing there watching me, looking at my big, jiggly butt and changing his mind.

*

I never did go and meet him, of course. When I got back to the house, my cousin noticed my deep blush and harassed me until I told her what had happened, at which point she continued to harass me to go and meet him, 'just for a coffee, a chat, but be careful because he's older'. I waffled all day about it, but in the end, I just couldn't do it. I kept picturing him sitting in the window, Al's head on his lap, looking up the street hopefully. But every time I had that pleasantly pathetic image in my mind, my cruel brain would replace it with a scene of him laughing and high-fiving with his friend about how he 'totally fucked with this fat high-school chick, and she'll be here any minute trying to get with me'. I tortured myself all day, alternating between the fantasy of him pining and what I told myself was the reality of him having played a cruel joke on a vulnerable teenage fatty.

In the end, I was trapped, immobilised between my desperate desire to be right to hope and my hopelessly ingrained cynicism and fear. My cousin, because she loved me and maybe because she forgot, dropped the subject eventually, and never brought it up again. But I never forgot about that boy, the only respectable boy ever to ask 'fat me' out. The only person who ever made me feel a spark of hope that being fat wasn't the end of the world, that maybe I could find someone decent, attractive, and my own age. That maybe someone *normal* could love me some day.

Up until that day, and that boy, my prospects had been limited to the fringes of society. There was the old drunk guy who smelled like piss and whisky, who grabbed my ass on his way onto the crowded bus and grazed my thigh on his way off, whispering 'Bye, sweet thing' into my ear. I was fifteen. Or there was the homeless man who worked the corner by my high school, who had one huge, matted dreadlock and a grin with more gaps than teeth, who used to call me 'baby' and ask me when I was going to marry him. And then there was that one nice nineteen-year-old boy who sat next to me on my bus home one day, who had some sort of mental disability, and who pulled the race card when I politely rejected his request for my phone number. I used his age as my excuse, but he didn't seem to be buying it, and it wouldn't have been politically correct to say: 'No, it's not because you're black, it's because you're *retarded*!'

Nobody else even looked twice at me, unless it was to ask for help with homework or request a recipe for madeleines or pass a message to my significantly cooler and more socially visible brother.

At first I told myself that my weirdness with guys – my

inability to flirt, my self-preserving instinct to act more like a guy than a girl – was the result of hitting puberty surrounded solely by other pubescent girls and old teacher-men. But it didn't get better, even after a year at high school, where I shared hallways, classrooms, and sometimes even eye contact with boys my age. I was still relegated, as I had been from an early age, to the Island of the Unfuckables. Anybody remotely normal or desirable immediately put me in the friend zone. The little-sister zone. The I'd-never-fuck-a-fatty zone.

I wasn't a sexual object. Not in my eyes, nor, it seemed, in anyone else's, besides the aforementioned homeless/drunk/disabled dudes and the one attractive, charming fluke I never had the guts to follow up on. I knew that fat girls in general could be loved – I'd seen them on the street or at the movies with dates, boyfriends, even husbands – and I even knew on some level that the hatred I harboured for my own fatness wasn't a requirement that all fat people followed. Once, in a random kitsch shop, I'd seen a fat-activism book, created from a zine, with pictures of fat bodies and funny stories about awkward fat moments in bed. It was called *Fat!So?* and it was all about how fat people are just people, and they can be healthy and sexual and funny, just as much as thin people can. I stood there and flipped through it, fascinated by the way these people felt about their large bodies – not just unashamed, but *proud* – but I didn't want to buy it. The only reason I took it home with me was because Andrea saw me reading it and insisted on getting it for me 'as a gift'. I knew she meant well, but I wasn't sure I wanted it. I wasn't even sure how I felt about it, besides a little uncomfortable and interested in a detached way.

I couldn't see how all that activism stuff applied to me. *Those* fat people might be proud and happy and in love, and I didn't begrudge them that, but neither did I relate. I was still trying to not *be* fat, so how could I join a movement that embraced it? I spent most of my time either on a diet or wilfully off it, eating all the 'bad' things I'd been denying myself while I was dieting. In those depressing moments when I had to admit to myself that I might never lose the weight, the absolute most I allowed myself to hope for romantically was that somebody could *see past* my body – that anybody could ever actually desire or love all 250+ pounds of me was beyond the realm of fantasy. And even though I felt strongly that nobody *would* ever like me enough to see past my body, I was embarrassingly vulnerable to suggestion. Any hint of something more than friendliness and I became infatuated with a guy. Any guy.

Chuck was the first; he was lanky and strange and wore black jeans and a dated leather jacket and practised karate moves in the hallway and said '*Gracias*' with a Castilian lisp that everyone in our Spanish class found really annoying and pretentious. I kept my freshman crush a secret for months before finally admitting it to my two best friends at my new school, Sara and Tessa, who teased me mercilessly for it. But they also must have recognised the dire limits of my potential dating pool, because they encouraged me to go eat pizza with him after school one day, which I did, at his invitation – that was the closest I got to going on a date my entire high-school career, and I could barely eat my slice of pizza because I was so nervous (not to mention hyper-conscious of eating unhealthy foods in front of a boy). Nothing ever came of it, and I grew to find Chuck more annoying than attractive. A couple of years later, he got a girlfriend from another school; she was fairly rotund herself, and if I hadn't changed my opinion about him by then I would have kicked myself for missing out on what might have actually been a possible relationship.

And then there was Alan. The Super-Jew. The politico. The only kid in the class who looked like he was forty and wore a yarmulke. He also wore Hawaiian shirts and khaki pants, and was obsessed with political history and terrible at writing essays. But he held doors and said things like 'Ladies first' and was probably the politest boy I'd ever met. And so, sophomore year, when a guy in our class told me Alan liked me, I scoffed and brushed it off, and then proceeded to feel something for him that I'd never experienced. More than a crush, more even than infatuation. What I felt for Alan was the closest I'd ever come to unrequited love. And, again, I told only my two best friends about my feelings. Tessa smiled gently and told me in an overly enthusiastic voice that Alan was 'really nice!' Sara nearly split her sides laughing at the thought that anybody would *like*-like Alan, and then started dating him the following year when he ditched the Hawaiian shirts and started playing soccer. They quickly became inseparable – we used to call them Saalan.

No matter how intensely I felt these crushes, I would never have dared to act on either of them. I wouldn't have known how. Boys were a whole different species to me: they were like pets, to be cared for and cooed over, or scolded and shooed off the sofa. The only boys I really observed closely were my brother and his friends, and if they weren't ignoring me they were usually either teasing me – his cute friend Yves used to ask me to have his babies and then laugh at my all-consuming blush – or worrying about me tattling – his even cuter friend Wilke walked into our kitchen once with a joint behind his ear and a forty-ounce of beer in his hand, saw me standing at the sink, and froze like he'd been busted by the cops. I was no more than a little sister, to be affectionately tortured or convinced not to snitch.

The Island of the Unfuckables is a lonely place. I spent evenings in my room, often crying or writing dramatic diary entries in which I bemoaned my fat, lonely lot in life (these were alternated with backtracking entries in which I bravely beat myself up for my self-absorbed whining and laid out a plan to lose weight). At school and with my friends, I pretended to be grown up and savvy about men and sex, but everything I said, the advice I gave with such confidence, came straight from the pages of *Cosmo* or from listening to my older brother and sister talk about their relationships. It was a farce, but it was a successful one; once, when I was sixteen, I met a girl who went to Courtney's artsy, alternative high school. We spent a few hours together, gossiping and chatting, and the girl later asked Courtney if I had a boyfriend. As if that were the most natural thing in the world, for a tubbo like me to be dating someone. Apparently she was shocked to learn that I'd never so much as held hands with a boy, much less kissed/fondled/screwed one. When Courtney told me that, I was thrilled. The ruse had worked!

But just because *she* believed I could have a boyfriend and a sex life, that didn't mean *I* believed it. And despite my slick trickery and humorous exterior, I was miserable inside. I hated to admit it to anyone except my diary, but I was really depressed. I spent hours lying on my bed, just staring at the wall and willing myself to cry, to scream, to do anything to expel the horrible sinking feeling in my chest that told me I would never lose weight, never find a boyfriend, and never be happy. Of course, I hid my depression extremely well – my unhappiness with my body and my perma-single status only ever came out in public as a self-deprecating joke, and I was good enough at those that people usually laughed instead of frowning concernedly.

Inside, though, when I allowed myself to face the gaping hole under my ribcage, I had to admit I was depressed and alone. I felt completely rejected by the world of boys. I was terrified that it was my destiny to be locked out of normal, dating society by my body – maybe I was meant to be fat, maybe it was in my genes, but if I wanted to get a boyfriend I knew I had to fight it. The only way I could think of to make it to the mainland from the Island was to lose weight, and now that there was more riding on it I tried even harder than I had before – a hundred different ways and a hundred different times. I tried diets – the cabbage soup diet, Atkins, Weight Watchers, no white foods, you name it – I went to Jazzercise with my mom and bought workout DVDs and went swimming at the YMCA on days when I trusted the pool to be empty, and I even went to weight-loss camp two summers in a row.

The camp was almost a fun way of losing weight; the other kids were fat too, so I felt like I fit in somehow (although of course there was a hierarchy dictated by just *how* fat each kid was). I made friends easily, and some of the girls even got boyfriends. But it wasn't exactly the 'normal' social life I'd been craving – it was more like being put in an enclosure with 'my own kind', like I was a chimp who'd tried to mix with humans, and now I was back with the chimps so I should have been happy to be socialising more easily. But what I wanted was to be *human*, even though I didn't see the other fat kids as inhuman somehow – just me. Despite being surrounded by people my size and bigger, I was still crippled by self-consciousness. Even if I wasn't the fattest girl in the pool at water aerobics class, I was still too fat to be in a swimsuit. Fat camp taught me that my own body issues had nothing to do with other people's bodies. It was all about me, and how much *I* hated me. If any guys were interested in me, I didn't notice; I was too busy hating myself and trying to convince myself that *this time* I would keep the weight off to pay any attention to boys. Anyway, paying attention to them would mean admitting to myself that I hoped for something, and at camp all my desperate hopes were pinned to weight loss. I didn't have any left over to spend on romance.

Although most of what I learned at camp was repetition of knowledge I'd already gained through years of dieting – lessons on portion control, calorie counting, good fats versus bad – the controlled environment and forced exercise made it easier to follow a routine without thinking so hard, and I dropped about twenty-five pounds my first summer. But just like everything I'd tried before, it ultimately failed; I gained it all back the following year. I was losing hope. Nothing I tried could make me feel like normalcy was within my grasp. I'd lose ten, fifteen, twenty pounds, and then the weight would dig its heels in and I'd give up. *If I can't even lose thirty pounds*, I'd think, *then why bother at all? Why torture myself when it's not going to do any good?* So I'd crash, and I'd go back to my bad habits: sneaking unhealthy food behind my mom's back; eating store-bought cookie dough instead of real food during my school lunch break; waiting for the bus to take me up our massive hill on the way home from school instead of just trudging up it with my backpack on, huffing and puffing be damned. And I not only gained back the weight I'd lost, I gained more, every time. I put on weight steadily, so you almost wouldn't notice if you saw me every day, but one day, all of a sudden, I crossed the line from fat to obese. I looked huge. Like a cartoon, or one of those people you see on the news stories about the Obesity Epidemic. No wonder boys didn't look twice at me: I was a monster.

Just like the boys, I was repulsed by me. I spent most of my time avoiding my body, doing my best to keep my eyes forward and my thighs covered. The last thing I wanted was to see myself. I would shower at ridiculous temperatures just to steam up the mirror so I didn't have to see my naked body when I got out. I never went to the beach or went tanning in Golden Gate Park with my high-school friends, prefer-ring the comforting dark of a movie theatre with Courtney or the anonymity of a long drive with Andrea in her par-ents' car. I tried my hardest not to look at myself, because when I did catch a glimpse of my hulking form, in a public restroom mirror or a glass storefront window, I crumbled in-side. Sometimes, if I was at home and I saw or felt a roll of chub, I would become fixated on it, pushing and pulling my belly and thighs and arms, desperately trying to rearrange the fat into some semblance of normality. It was safer for me to avoid my body than to confront it, because confronting it always led to tears and despondence, and more than once it even led to bruising.

I hated myself for failing to lose the weight. I couldn't un-derstand why it was so hard for me, and yet at the same time, I did understand that the 'why' didn't matter: it *was* hard, and the only way I would be able to change my body would be to have the willpower to control what I put into it. But I couldn't. I tried and tried and tried, and failed every time, and I despised myself for my weakness. I was desperate.

If someone had offered me a trade, my soul or my first-born or even a few decades of my life in exchange for a normal body, I would have taken it in an instant. Because on a very private level, deep beneath the flesh that tormen-ted me, I *was* normal. I was just another teenage girl, and I wanted the same things every teenage girl wants: a hand to hold, someone to text and giggle over, someone to make me feel like a woman instead of a little kid. And every time I realised this desire would never be fulfilled, I broke a little bit more, until I was so depressed I could barely see straight. Until I was thinking about suicide, holding debates with myself over the pros and cons (pros: no more crying, no more pain, no more *fat*; cons: my family will be destroyed, I'll never see my friends again, my family will be destroyed). Until I was so desperate I sometimes thought I'd never make it through high school alive.

And then, one day in the summer before my junior year, when I was sixteen, I read an article in the *New Yorker*, and for the first time in years everything felt . . . *possible*.

4

San Francisco, July 2001

I drop my heavy bag on the floor, kick off my flip-flops, and walk into the living room without looking up from the magazine I found on the doormat. I check the table of contents and turn to page 69, sit down on the sofa and start reading, ignoring the afternoon light slanting through the big living-room picture window and the sun twinkling on the Bay Bridge outside, disregarding my need to pee and my thirst for something cold. I don't stop until I reach the end – I even skip all the cartoons on the corners of the pages.

The 'Annals of Science' section of the *New Yorker* magazine isn't really my thing. I usually just flip through and read the funnies, standing in the hall with my backpack still on, then drop the magazine back on the table where I found it and go upstairs to my room. Sometimes, when I've settled into the quiet of evening, I'll read the fiction piece, but more often I just skim the 'Shouts and Murmurs' and then go back to the latest Margaret Atwood novel or whatever other book I've currently got my nose in day and night. But this week's issue has an article that's grabbed my attention.

It's about something called gastric bypass surgery, a relatively new, controversial procedure to force obese bodies to lose a large amount of weight, often over a hundred pounds, very quickly. Surgeons cut away a tiny section of the stomach (about the size of a thumb!) and make another division in the small intestine, about 18 inches down. Then they rearrange the whole mess so the patient ends up with a teeny stomach, leading directly to a later part of the intestine (bypassing the rest of the stomach and the section of intestine that digests fats and sugars). They reattach that bit further down, so the whole thing ends up looking like a sort of squishy Y-formation.

It's seen as a last resort for the morbidly obese: surgery is the *only* treatment for obesity that has been found to be consistently effective. The article investigates the surgery and deems it strange – it doesn't treat any specific disease or repair an injury, it is simply a medical control of people's will – and very possibly a breakthrough in the fight against obesity, but the writer also points out that the procedure is risky and dangerous. One in two hundred patients dies as a result of the surgery, and one in ten suffers serious complications such as infection or blood clots.

But I don't care about that. My heart is racing; my eyes can hardly digest the words on the page fast enough. One thing runs through my mind, and one thing only: *this is it*. All I can see in the lines of journalistic objectivity is possibility; to me, this surgery is the Holy Grail I never knew to search for. When I've finished the article, I go back over the most exciting bits, my lips moving and trembling as I read: 'most patients . . . lose at least two thirds of their excess weight (generally more than a hundred pounds) within a year'; 'ten-year follow-up studies find an average regain of only ten to twenty pounds'; 'the gastric bypass is the one thing . . . that works.'*

When I've calmed down a bit and my legs feel less shaky, I stand up and set the magazine on the coffee table, folded open to the article – the title, 'The Man Who Couldn't Stop Eating', blaring across the top and a brightly coloured illustration of a thin man inside layers of fat on the facing page. I'm praying that the piece will plant the same seed in my dad that it's planted in me, and share with him the tender hope that's already uncoiling its leaves in my heart.

When he gets home an hour later I'm upstairs in my room, trying and failing to focus on my book while dreams of normalcy drift through my mind. The old walls of our house rattle as he slams the door and bellows his usual 'Hellooooo?' Mom has gone straight from doing the books at Catie's flower store to her Jazzercise class – she won't be home for another couple of hours. It's just us. I call a hello back to him, then hold my breath as I wait the twenty minutes I figure it'll take him to look in the fridge, pull a grape or two off the bunch on the kitchen counter, leaving the little nubs of bare stem that drive my mom mad, then make his way to the sofa and my carefully set trap.

'Hey.' I try to sound casual as I saunter into the kitchen, avoiding his line of sight. He doesn't respond – a good sign.

---

* *New Yorker*, 9 July 2001, pp. 72–5.

I peer around the corner into the living room. Yep, he's reading it. Giddy and anxious, I grab a string cheese from the fridge and tiptoe back up to my room. I try again to read, but I can't even absorb a sentence without having to go back over it – my brain is impervious to anything but this new idea. So I just listen. When I hear him moving around again I get up and clomp down the stairs. This time I go through the living room first – yes, the magazine is closed now, thrown haphazardly onto the sofa. I continue into the kitchen.

'Hey, kiddo.' Dad closes the fridge door. 'How you doin'?'

'OK. You?' I open the fridge door as he shifts back over to the fruit bowl. *Nope, still nothing tempting in the fridge.* I can tell my dad is disappointed with the lack of snackables too. He looks up from the grapes with a sigh.

'Yeah, all right. Your mom at her class?'

'Yep.'

We're silent for a moment as we graze, the two of us moving awkwardly around each other in the small room like a pair of Cape buffalo. He opens the pantry door and I think about going upstairs and rooting through my backpack for something more satisfying, but instead I steel my nerves and get right to the point.

'Hey, did you see the new *New Yorker*?'

'Yup.'

'There was an interesting article in it . . .'

'The one about the surgery? Hey, sign us *up*, huh?' His hands come up to shoulder level and form into double thumbs-up as his face breaks into an excited grin.

I laugh, trying to pretend this is just another conversation for me, like this will be all his idea.

'I know, right?'

We're quiet again, and then I can't take it any more. *Is he really going to breeze past this opportunity?* I can't let that happen. I bite the bullet.

'Um, Dad? Really? Sign us up?'

He turns away from the grapes and looks at me. My face is burning so hot I'm afraid it might start sweating. He cocks his head, frowns a little, then nods slowly.

'OK. I'll have my assistant look into it.'

I swallow, and nod, then disappear back into my room. Now all that's left is to wait and see if he follows through.

Almost six months later, just a week after my seventeenth birthday, I lay out my flesh on a cold slab and count backwards from ten.

*

Both my dad and I had been gaining weight steadily. In the six years since we'd moved from Manhattan Beach and I'd gotten serious about watching my weight, I had nonetheless gone from fearing the two-hundred-pound mark to flying past it and refocusing my fear on the 250 mark; now, at 290 pounds, I was terrified of hitting the three-hundred-pound, no-denying you're not just fat but morbidly obese point. Although I'd tried diets and gimmicks and camps and personal trainers, I hadn't made any significant progress – I could lose fifteen or thirty pounds if I really set my mind to it, but I always gained it back, plus more – and although Dad had talked about trying a million diets and gimmicks, he always slid pretty quickly back into rich business dinners and keeping bowls of jelly beans on his desk. It was clear to both of us that this was our big chance. Times had gotten desperate, and desperate measures were now called for.

Of course, simply making the decision to have surgery, to risk our lives for a chance at normalcy, wasn't all there was to it.

Financially, I was incredibly lucky – all those long, jelly-bean-fuelled hours and high-calorie business dinners meant my dad could afford to pay out of pocket for both of our surgeries, no small matter since each cost upwards of $25,000, not including the cost of flights to San Diego, hotel stays, and medications, and that was with a discount for paying cash – it was tricky getting insurance to cover it in those days. We would both go through the procedures at the same time, which meant I didn't need to remind him of my desperate desire, or worse, nag him to do the administration required – once my dad has his mind made up, pretty much nothing can stop him. But if I thought that all I had to sort out was money and logistics, I was sorely mistaken.

First, there was the conversation with my mom, who didn't seem to mind that I'd hoped my dad would take care of everything, but who also didn't fully support the idea of an 'easy out'. My mom's a tough bird – she believes in working hard for what you want, and fighting your own battles without help. I got the feeling that she wished I would wait a while; I was still so young, and had so much time to try to change my habits and turn my life around. But from my point of view, I had my whole life ahead of me, and the sooner I got to live that life as a normal person, the better. I'd be off to college in two years, and if I had this surgery maybe I could start over then. We didn't talk about it as much or as intimately as most mothers and daughters probably would – my mom was never the type to be very comfortable with conversations about emotions or personal demons – but we talked until we understood each other. I felt like she would never fully understand why I had to have surgery just to lose weight, or even why I had gained so much weight in the first place, and I soon learned that I would have to face the fact that neither would a lot of others. People would always look at me and wonder why I had surgery instead of just *not eating so much*. But my mom had known me my whole life, had watched me try and fail to control my weight a million times, and she was no dummy – I think on some level she must have known that this was the only way to stop the ever-increasing waistbands of her husband and daughter. Lord knows *she'd* done everything she could. So, however reluctantly, she agreed to come with us to an information session in Mountain View, about a forty-minute drive south of San Francisco.

For an hour or so, we sat in a conference room at the Hyatt hotel with about fifty other desperate strangers, their (and our) massive bottoms overhanging the narrow straight-backed chairs, as we all listened to a panel of doctors from the Alvarado Hospital for Bariatric Medicine in San Diego discuss the details of the surgery, the costs, the benefits, and the dangers. They told us if we went through the surgery we could expect to get very ill every time we ate fatty or sugary foods, and we would be in real pain if we overate. It was a serious decision, and they urged us to think very carefully about whether it was the right choice for us. '*Blah blah blah* . . .' Again, I glazed over when they started talking about the reality of post-surgery life, the complications and risks involved – I just wanted to get to the good part, where they'd promise us we'd lose the weight and tell us stories of people who had the surgery and got to live the life they'd always dreamed of. I felt like I'd understood all the medical mumbo-jumbo from reading the article and looking at the diagram of the surgery, and none of that was important to me at all. After so long spent hating myself, hating the fleshy body I felt so trapped in, I was ready to start hoping again. This was the first time in years that I could feel the optimism blooming in the cave in my chest, and that was all I could focus on. All the other stuff was just noise.

When the meeting was over, and I was one step closer to my own personal salvation, we had dinner across the parking lot at Sizzler's, a chain fish restaurant that I'd only ever seen commercials for. Under normal circumstances, Mom would never have allowed us to eat at the kind of place where damn near everything was battered and fried, but it was getting late and restaurant chains were all we could see nearby. It *was* Mountain View, after all; we couldn't expect our usual standard of dinner options in a suburb. Over battered shrimp and butter-slathered steak, Dad chattered excitedly about how we'd never be able to eat like this again after the surgery. I nodded, although it was hard to imagine being unable to eat more than a fist-sized portion of anything before I felt full, and actually getting sick from fat and sugar. But I didn't care what we could or couldn't put into our bodies, as long as it didn't require constant vigilance and willpower and the dark, lurking knowledge of failure to come. I was happy to live the rest of my life unable to eat fried things without getting sick; I just wanted to be thin. I didn't care what my future diet would consist of, so long as the restrictions were placed on me by my *body*, rather than the miserable process of using my mind to exert willpower over my desires and desperately trying to hold out hope that this time it would actually get somewhere, while battling with the near-certainty that even if I did lose weight, it wouldn't be enough and I'd gain it all back anyway. It was exhausting just thinking about going through that all over again; I wanted to focus instead on trying to imagine what it might be like to lose the weight. I'd been fat for so long by that point that I could hardly picture myself with a normal body – my dad had spent a good portion of his life as a fit, athletic, normal-sized person, but as long as I could remember I'd been at best chubby and at worst morbidly obese. Now I barely touched my food, my stomach churning with anxiety and excitement as visions of normal-sized clothing and loose wrist bangles danced in my head. Mom just picked at her limp salad and looked anxious.

When we got back to the city, my parents sat down and had a serious discussion about just how to proceed. If it were only my dad having the surgery, it probably wouldn't have been such a big deal, but my age complicated things. I was still only sixteen, so my parents would have to give legal consent to the surgery for me. Not only that, but the doctors at the centre were hesitant as well; the surgery was a relatively new tactic, and although they had had plenty of practice, it wasn't commonplace for them to perform it on young patients. I think I was one of the first few, in fact. Much to my teenage dismay, I discovered that if I wanted my miracle solution, I was going to have to jump through some hoops. The doctors required a psychological evaluation to make sure I could handle the stresses and changes the surgery would bring about, and my parents added their own stipulation: I would have to see the therapist for a full year, starting as soon as possible and finishing the summer after the operation. I was angry – the thought of talking to a stranger about my feelings made me feel humiliated before I even began, besides which I couldn't imagine any *negative* emotional effects that would result from losing weight – but I agreed. There were physical assessments to pass too: glucose tolerance, all kinds of endocrinal tests, a very involved examination ... it felt like a never-ending process, but I was determined to see this one through. I was convinced it was the only way to allow me to eat like a normal person without always watching myself, berating myself, associating everything I put in my mouth with a feeling of pride or guilt or shame – I wanted food to be just *food*, what it was to naturally thin people, instead of it always being a threat or a forbidden desire or a disappointment. So I gritted my teeth and went along with everything the doctors and my parents required (at least on the surface – during my first few months in therapy, I got so good at misdirecting with comments about politics or the weather that I could have taught Siegfried and Roy a thing or two).

Once the tests and evaluations were out of the way, and my dad's assistant had managed to schedule us for back-to-back surgeries just after Christmas, I had to start telling people. I figured it was better to tell my friends before I stopped eating and started throwing up a lot and losing weight really fast, just to limit how freaked out they'd get. And also for my own sake, I wanted to rip the Band-Aid off quickly and painfully, rather than stretching the awkwardness out over months. So I gathered my eight closest girlfriends in my room and blurted out the news. They took it as well as a group of sixteen-year-olds can be expected to take such intense news, and nearly all of them were extremely supportive.

Next came family. Andrew, a mini-Dad when it came to uncomfortable conversations or long goodbyes, brushed off the news with a vague comment of support – 'Awesome, dude, whatever makes you guys happy.' My more extended family, cousins and aunts, I left to my mom. So that was everybody told, phew. Except it wasn't – there was one more person to tell, and I was *not* looking forward to it.

I had expended a lot of energy in recent years avoiding talking to Catie about my weight. She was naturally slender, despite her constant buddy-diets with my mom and her complaints about fifteen pounds here or a size 10 pair of jeans there, and she couldn't understand why I was the way I was. And it's not as if I knew how to explain it to her – hell, I couldn't fully explain it to myself. Even when I did allow myself a bit of introspection, some level of investigation into why I was fat (especially when my siblings weren't), I never figured it out. I circled around the potential reasons in my own mind – *Dad's fat too, so it must be linked to genes; I really like sweets and don't stick to diets for long enough, so it probably is all my fault; I'm not good at sports, and I don't like the gym, so even though I walk a lot I'm not active enough to ever burn off all this excess* – but I could never arrive at any sort of logical conclusion. I had friends who ate much worse than I did, who never moved from their sofas unless forced, and who would have fit in one leg of my jeans, with room to spare. Thinking about why I was fat was confusing and depressing – I usually just ended up beating myself up and feeling even worse about myself than I already did, which wasn't exactly a great motivator to fight the flab – so I didn't do it often. In the end, the only real answer I ever got from these brief, miserable moments of consideration was that it didn't matter. It didn't matter how I got there, I *was* there, and what mattered now was figuring out how to get out. And until the surgery presented itself as an option, I couldn't see any exits from where I stood, which is exactly why I had avoided the topic of my weight at all costs, especially with my sister, who pursued it more belligerently than anyone else in my life. The few times we *had* discussed my increasing girth, she'd sat me down and cried while telling me she was worried about me. I believed her, but really, is there anything worse to a fifteen-year-old fatty than having her normal-sized sister crying at her about how she needs to lose weight?

So I put off telling her – put it off for months. She knew about my dad's surgery months ahead of time – he'd never been one for keeping secrets – but I hadn't found the right time to tell her that I would be joining him under the knife. Until the time found me, on Christmas Eve, three days before the surgery. I don't know if I would *ever* have told her, if Andrew hadn't blurted out something about it in front of her. Oh, man, did I wish I'd told her earlier, because the consequence of my reluctance was an extremely uncomfortable half hour of her crying in my room about how I could keep something this important from her. I wanted to go under anaesthesia right then.

But that was pretty much the worst of it, at least emotionally. The next day, my parents and I flew to San Diego – my mom wedged into the middle seat between us for what I'm sure she hoped would be the last time – and checked into our hotel for the two weeks we'd have to stay in town. Then shit got real, fast. There was the physical, including a rectal exam (which has to be every seventeen-year-old's nightmare, whether she's skinny or fat). There was a mandatory support-group session in a grey room, too small to comfortably hold all of the huge women in sweat suits and twinsets spilling over the sides of their chairs. And me, folding inward and politely nodding as they all blubbered in my direction about how lucky I was to be doing this so early on in my life's journey (I never thought I'd be willing to trade something for another rectal exam). And then, finally, there was the day of reckoning, which involved a lot of nudity, poking, prodding, and waiting around.

I was up early the day of surgery, to get to the hospital around 7 a.m. for prepping. I had to get completely naked, put on an open-backed hospital gown and some surprisingly cosy compression socks, sign a bunch of forms, be weighed and measured and given an IV (in my hand, because my arm was too fat to find a vein), get into the bed, be covered with blankets, and then . . . wait. I couldn't believe how long I had to sit there in the bed, waiting. And the longer I waited, the more I thought: about how scared I was to go under anaesthesia; about how badly I wanted this to be the last 'lifestyle change' I had to try; and about whether the doctors would be able to perform the surgery laparoscopically, as planned, or whether my organs would prove too big for them to see around with the scope, in which case they'd have to slice me right down the middle of my belly.

It had been two days of this shit; more people had seen me naked and learned my weight in the past twelve hours than the past twelve years. I'd worked hard to make sure those things stayed hidden, and now they were everybody's business – I was anxious to make them history instead of fact. Not to mention that I hadn't even had a sip of water since midnight, so the thought of even an hour extra made me want to give up and go drink a breakfast shake. I toughed it out, though – I'd come this far and been fat for this long, and I figured I could wait a bit longer. Anyway, the doctor would get there soon and they'd put me under and that would be the end of it.

But it would also be the chance for a new beginning, a new life with a new body and, hopefully, a new body image.

My mom's hand is dry and warm on mine. I look down at the white hospital sheet and see our hands, mine as puffy and pink as always, fingernails short and blunt, and hers small, slender, the skin tanned and slightly spotted from the sun. I try to remember the last time we held hands, try to focus on the sensation of her index finger stroking the skin around my IV tube.

I look up at her face; it's drawn with worry. We've been waiting here since 7 a.m. I'm exhausted – I barely slept last night, kept awake by nerves and thirst. And now that we're here, and I've put on the gown and taken off all my jewellery and had an IV put into the back of my hand (and managed not to cry as the nurse stabbed over and over, unable to find a vein for what felt like decades), they're not ready for us. My mom sees me looking at her and manages a smile.

'Don't worry, Anna,' she says, 'it'll be over soon.'

To the nurse who has come to check on us, she says: 'Can't you at least get her something for her nerves?'

The nurse comes back and attaches something to my IV, and soon I feel the vice around my heart start to ease.

'It'll all be over soon,' my mom says again, patting the backs of my fingers to avoid jostling the tube.

*

'Well, hey there, Anne!' *The doctor comes striding into the room looking way too perky for my liking. I remind myself that perky is good; he is, after all, about to slice me open and rearrange my insides. I smile feebly at him.*

'OK, Anne, now I know Dr E. told you she wasn't feeling one hundred per cent after she finished your dad's surgery, so she called me in.'

I nod. My mom is with my dad right now, waiting for him to wake up. She said she'd be back before I went in, though.

'Well I just want you to know that even though it's my day off, I'm one hundred and ten per cent ready to do your surgery, and you're in good hands. OK?' He gives my shoulder a squeeze and grins down at me. I just nod again.

The doctor heads off to scrub up, and I take huge breaths to calm my racing pulse. I had only just gotten comfortable with Dr E. – despite being slender, blonde, and pretty, she had turned out to be pretty cool – when she came into my room to tell me she wasn't going to be performing my surgery. I like this guy less, mostly just because he's a man and I don't particularly want him seeing me naked, but he is the head of Bariatric Medicine, so I guess he must be good.

I take another deep breath and watch the door for my mom. She should be back any minute. Don't forget, *I tell myself,* to them, you're just a big slab of meat. Like a cow to a butcher

– they aren't judging, they're just looking for the best place to slice you open.

My mom is back. She says my dad is doing fine, if a bit groggy. She, too, squeezes my shoulder, but less aggressively than the doctor. Her squeeze actually makes me feel a bit better. If my dad is fine, then I will be too.

The doctor pops his head around the doorframe.

'Ready, Anne?'

I swallow, my throat dry, and try to smile. No, *I think,* no, *no, I'm not ready at all. But I nod anyway.*

Two orderlies come into the room and station themselves one on either side of my bed. The nurse grabs my IV and they all work together to wheel my bed away from the wall. As we pass my mom, she gives my arm a quick stroke and tells me she'll be here when I wake up. I want to tell her I love her, but I'm afraid of not being stoic enough, so I just nod. Again. My neck is starting to get tired.

I rest my head back on the pillow and watch the ceiling tiles slide past.

*

The operating room is cold. I feel my nipples harden against the cotton gown and I blush, remembering how naked I am under the blankets. The bed stops moving and I look around; there are machines everywhere, with cords hanging off them and big, wide screens with numbers and symbols I don't understand. There are more people than I expected in here. One of the young men has come over to help the orderlies.

'OK, Anne,' he says, his voice kinder than I expected, 'don't move, OK? Just let us take care of you.'

He looks at the other two guys and nods. They grip the sheet beneath me. I try not to tense my body, but I can't help holding my breath.

'On three,' he says. 'One, two, three!'

I feel the sheet tighten under me and my body slides easily over onto the operating table. I'm surprised: I had braced myself for the awkward moment when they couldn't lift me and I had to crawl over on my own, shaky and massive like a newborn walrus. I hardly have time to register my new location before they're piling me with warm, heavy blankets and tucking me in.

'Hi, Anne,' another new face appears next to me. Another man, this one a bit older than the others, maybe mid-forties. 'I'm Dr J., I'm your anaesthesiologist today. I'm just going to gently put you to sleep now, and we're going to take real good care of you, OK?'

Another masculine shoulder squeeze. Another nod.

'Now, Anne, I'm going to need you to count backwards from ten for me, OK?'

I clear my throat. 'OK.' It feels strange to speak. My mouth is so dry.

'Ten, nine . . .' I feel like an idiot, counting out loud while people bustle all around me. It's not going to work anyway, *I* think, *I don't feel sleepy at all.*

'Eight, seven . . .' My eyes droop, and before I can say 'six' the room has gone dark.

II

AFTER

5

San Diego, California, January 2002

I glower at my chicken noodle soup. My mom and my aunt Nancy are eating their solid meals happily, picking out the bits they like best and leaving everything else sitting on the dull white deli plates. I look across the table at my dad, who's frowning down at his own bowl of clear broth with off-limits chunks of carbs, chicken and vegetables. He sighs, picks up his spoon, and skims some liquid off the top, blowing on it a little. He sips the broth off the spoon, then sets it back down on the plate under the shadow of the bowl. He looks exhausted, as if that one little motion has wiped him out for the day. I know how he feels.

It's been a week since we had our surgeries. After two days in the hospital, in a painkiller haze punctuated by nurses bustling in and out and my mom going from my room to my dad's and back again, we all moved to the Residence Inn, where we're staying in a suite for two weeks. It has two bedrooms, a living room, and a small kitchen where my mom can make our endless 'meals' of chicken broth and/or sugar-free Jell-O. Today is the first time Dad and I have left the hotel – Mom has gotten out for at least an hour most days, sometimes making up errands just to get a break from the oppressive post-op atmosphere.

I don't blame her. I've been going stir-crazy in there too. I thought two weeks of watching TV and relaxing would be great, but by the second day I wanted to rip my stitches just for something to do. I think Mom could tell, because she's planned this little outing today, and she's put up with us like a champ, despite our groans of pain every time the car hits a pothole or we have to move our abdomens more than an inch. Considering how much she hates playing nurse, she's been pretty good so far.

She's delighted now to be out in the world, among the living. I watch her across the table, talking with her older sister, her best friend, and I realise I haven't seen her smile all week until now. Her face has either been scrunched in worry or slack with exhaustion. I feel a pang of guilt, mingled with resentment. The usual reaction.

'Anna, eat your soup.'

My mom has caught me looking at her, and paused her conversation to fuss over me. The past week has been an anomaly in my life: my mom and doctors worrying that I'm not eating *enough*, for once. I'm just so sick to death of broth and Jell-O, and when you add that to the swollen pain inside my stomach, under my luckily tiny scars, I don't exactly thrill at the idea of mealtimes.

I stare down at my soup again. I've had a few sips of the broth, and thank God it's homemade; any more of the canned stuff and I just might go on a hunger strike. I smile slightly at the irony of the thought. *Isn't that kind of the point of this surgery*, I think, *a forced hunger strike? Taking a stand against fat, without having to carry the sign and walk the picket line myself?*

I dip the spoon in the soup, watching the pale yellow liquid spill over the silvery edges and into the concave centre. A carrot slips in, and I move to put it back into the bowl and get another scoop of just broth, but then I pause. I look up – Mom and Nancy are chatting again, and Dad is leaning back in his chair with his eyes closed, a grimace on his face. I glance back at the carrot.

How bad could it possibly be? I mean, if I mush it up really well, it's gotta be about the same consistency as Jell-O, right?

I look around again, check that the coast is still clear, and then I quickly pop the spoon into my mouth. I swallow the broth, leaving the carrot sitting on my tongue. My heart beats a little faster. It's been days since I've put anything solid in my mouth.

Slowly, carefully, I raise my tongue and press the carrot against the roof of my mouth. It's soft, and small pieces break off the edges and slide down the sides of my tongue. The flavour is amazing: sweet, a little bit salty, fresh but mild. I never want to stop eating this carrot; what I really want is to chew it, to use my teeth again, but I don't dare let my parents see my jaw working, and anyway the thing is already mush. Too soon, I've swallowed, and the experience is over.

Without the ecstasy of texture to distract me, I start to

stress out. My face gets hot and my heart beats faster as the fear that maybe I've done something terrible takes over. I calm myself down by breathing deeply; I pay close attention to my insides, imagine I can feel the orange mush sliding down my throat toward that swollen opening to my new stomach – *OK, so far, so good.* Emboldened, I dip the spoon again, this time 'accidentally' catching a bit of celery. The worry is replaced again by delight as I mash the vegetable against my palate, revelling in the flavour of something different, green and refreshing; I've never found celery as exciting as I do today. I reach for another bite – *bite, bite! I finally get to bite something!*

'Anna?'

I drop the spoon into the bowl a little too quickly and look up. My mom is giving me a quizzical look.

'Yeah? What?'

'Are you ready? *The Royal Tenenbaums* starts in fifteen minutes.'

Shit. Shit! I feel panicked, and look down at my soup like it's a loved one from which I'm about to be separated.

'Uh, OK, I'm just –'

'Well, finish your broth if you want. The theatre's only across the way.'

My mom must be really pleased to see me interested in food if she's willing to be less than early. But they're all watching me now – there's no way I'll get another solid bit in.

I sigh, pick up the bowl, and slurp the broth off the top, looking cross-eyed down my nose at all those wasted chunks of texture and taste. I feel a bit like crying as I set it down and look up at my family. They're waiting for me, trying not to rush me, encouraging me with their eyes. I just want them to go away so I can break the rules in peace. I push my chair back from the table and begin the slow process of standing up.

'OK, let's go, I'm done.'

As we make our deliberate, painful way over to the theatre, my aunt falls in beside me. I look up at her from my hunched position and try to smile. She touches my arm.

'How are you feeling? Really?'

Tears prick the edges of my eyes but I grin through them, hoping my overenthusiasm will make them go away. If there's anyone I could really talk to about all the thoughts tangling themselves in my mind right now – the concern about the pain; the visions of what I might look like if I get thin; the desire to chew something solid; the hope that it'll be worth it; the fear that, just like every other weight-loss method I've tried, this one will fail (*I'll* fail, again) and I'll stay fat – it would be my aunt. She's always been a bit of an anomaly in her family: emotionally available, nurturing, *sweet*. We all call her Nancy Nurse, because she's the person you go to if you need a sympathetic pat or a years-old-still-good codeine pill. But I stop myself from telling her how I really feel. I'm afraid if I allow anyone access to the jumble, I'll also have to start trying to untangle it myself. So instead I keep smiling.

'Yeah, OK. I mean, it hurts, and I'm *really* sick of Jell-O, but other than that it's OK. It's just nice to be out of the house!'

My aunt puts her arm around my shoulder and gives it a gentle squeeze, and we continue on in silence. As I waddle along, my tongue probes the insides of my mouth for leftover bits of carrot or celery, and my eyes rove upward, over the long, lithe body of Gwyneth Paltrow on the movie poster, and my brain tangles itself even further.

*

The first thing people asked me when I went back to school was whether recovering from the surgery was painful, and it was, but mostly it was just *boring*. Spending two weeks unable to move much may have sounded like a great forced vacation, but the reality of it was cabin fever. As much as I hated my body, I also learned how much I'd taken it for granted – it may have been gross and embarrassing, but it functioned surprisingly well, and I'd never fully appreciated it for that. After a few days of Oprah and *Days of Our Lives* I would have killed for a walk around the block.

The recovery was also awkward. It's always embarrassing being poked and prodded, having doctors all up in your business, but when the business involves intestines that means rectal exams and questions about poop and all kinds of stuff that would make normal teenagers want to die on the spot, let alone an obese teen who's already so self-conscious it's almost painful to look at her. For example, I never knew anything about suppositories until the operation, and once we were introduced all I knew was that I never wanted to experience them again. That first meeting, two weeks after the surgery, was burned into my memory.

Picture (or better yet, don't) a 260-pound seventeen-year-old on her knees and elbows on the bathroom floor, trying to insert a suppository so she can have a bowel movement and get the all-clear from the doctors to go home and die of shame. In the end, I wasn't sure the medicine had worked, but I told my parents it had. I lied like my life depended on it, and I was allowed to fly back to San Francisco the next day. Lying to my doctors about something as important as whether my intestines were working properly was probably one of the stupider things I'd ever done, but I was desperate. I needed, more than anything, to be done with bodies and butts and poop and prodding. *Just get me home*, that was all I could think as I lay on the bathroom floor, the tears rolling down my fat, exhausted face.

That's not to say that the recovery was only about boredom and emotional discomfort. It *was* painful, a deep, gut-wrenching pain any time I moved or laughed or breathed. But we were lucky to have had the surgery through three small incisions in the skin, meaning we didn't have big, long wounds that would take longer to heal and would leave nasty scars. The pain was mostly interior, and the worst of that was controlled by Vicodin by the end of the first week – anyway, it was pretty easy to distract myself from the pain with thoughts of the coming thinness. Every time I felt a sharp twinge in my abdomen, I would revel in it a little bit; after all, 'no pain, no gain', right? So if there was that much pain, I figured, I had a lot to gain (or lose, as the case would

hopefully be). I spent most of my time laid up on the couch
or in bed trying to imagine myself as a thin person, or even
just a normal person: I stared at my wrists and tried to picture the knob of bone sticking out the way it did on my
mom's arms; I ran my hands over the mound of my belly and
imagined a flat plane instead; I lifted one leg in the air and
envisioned it looking long and lean, like Catie's. When I got
super absorbed in my fantasies, I didn't even notice that my
body hurt. Until I moved. But the pain, while significant,
was manageable with this combination of medication and
imagination. The more pressing physical difficulty had to do
with eating.

There was a reason we were on a strict regimen of broth
and Jell-O and the odd scrambled egg for the first two
weeks: our stomachs had gone through major trauma.
When the doctors isolated the section of the organ that
would become our permanently smaller stomachs (over
ninety per cent smaller than they were when we went in),
they also made the opening from that little pouch to the
intestine really small. This was intentional; by making it
harder for food to flow through our systems, the doctors
made the process slower, which in turn meant we should stay
'fuller' longer and feel more satisfied.

That's all fine and dandy, but when your stomach is
swollen from the damage of surgery *on top of* being made to
be teeny when the swelling subsides, that makes for a seriously uncomfortable first step in the digestive process. The
swelling didn't go down significantly for at least a month,
and it was probably another month before I learned to chew

my food until it could be pushed through a sieve. Which meant a good two months of vomiting after the majority of my meals, because when it can't go down, it's got to come back up.

It got pretty bad back at school, only two and a half weeks after the operation. My good friends knew about it, but I still wanted to act like nothing was different, so although I ate less at lunch and avoided fatty and sugary foods, I wasn't as careful as I should have been about chewing well. Not only was swallowing improperly chewed food *extremely* painful (like trying to get down a swallowful of jagged rocks) but it wasn't always successful. Sometimes, especially if I'd eaten in a hurry and then rushed to class, I had to excuse myself and go throw up in the bathroom. Most people probably didn't notice – high school is by its nature populated by narcissists – but a couple of my less close friends did, the ones who didn't merit advance warning but cared enough about me to wonder why my eyes were always watery when I got back from the bathroom after lunch. They may also have wondered if my suddenly baggy jeans had any connection to those watery eyes; I'd lost thirty pounds in the first two weeks after surgery, and the weight kept dropping off once I'd moved on to more solid foods (partly because, after a couple of months of everything I ate making me throw up, very little appealed to me any more).

My classmate Debbie was the first to ask. She sat down next to me during art class, after one particularly bad post-lunch bathroom run, and asked me whether I was OK. I was surprised at the genuine concern in her face; Debbie was one of the 'popular clique', and while I'd always liked her, I never thought anybody who could be best friends with the stereotypical 'queen bee' could possibly give me a second glance. But I told her the truth. She frowned through my explanation, and when I finished she just said:

'Oh, thank God. I thought you were bulimic or something.'

I never regretted telling Debbie about my surgery, but I was still wary of spilling the beans to anyone and everyone. I'd made a deal with myself: if you're going to do it, you can't hide it – no shame, or else you shouldn't have done it in the first place. But the truth is, it's hard to tell people that you've had elective surgery. Whether it's a gastric bypass or a nose job, the fear of judgement is very real.

And it wasn't just that; telling people something so intimate created a bridge between them and me. This wasn't always a bad thing. When I'd known someone for a while and I felt like the friendship could develop, I would often bring up the GB myself. It was important for my friends to understand what I'd been through and who I was. But occasionally people I wasn't so close to would ask questions, and then I'd have to choose before I was ready – did I tell them and risk an intimacy that neither of us was ready for, or did I fib or deflect, thus breaking my pact with myself to always be honest about my experience? It was an awkward place to be.

In the months before the GB, my dad and I had gone to multiple information sessions, designed to prepare us for what was to come: the surgery itself, the recovery pain, and the restrictions of life after we'd healed. Most importantly, we learned the four rules of a post-GB life:

Protein first: Always eat the protein on your plate first. Protein should make up eighty per cent of each meal, in order to help your bones and muscles stay strong as you go into what is essentially starvation mode, and you don't want to fill up on other stuff before you can get your protein in.

Drink your water: To flush your body of ketones as you drop weight very quickly, drink at least eight cups of water a day.

No snacking: The easiest way to gain back all the weight you lose with GB is to eat a *lot* of little meals, thus consuming thousands of extra calories despite your small stomach and difficulties with fat and sugar.

Exercise every day: You need to keep your muscles strong while you're losing weight and make sure it's just fat that's burned off by the body's caloric-stressed panic.

They warned us about throwing up, and told us horror stories about 'dumping syndrome', the newly rearranged intestines' reaction to sugars and fats, which involves feeling really dizzy and horrible and then getting awful diarrhoea. We heard positive tales of new love and old love rekindled after weight loss, and *you-go-girl* stories of women who lost the weight and divorced their loser husbands. I was repeatedly informed of the increase in fertility that accompanies a drop in body-fat percentage (my reaction: if anybody wanted to have sex with me, do you think I'd *be here*?). We even heard about people who lost so much excess weight that their skin sagged, empty and flaccid, and they had to have plastic surgery to tighten it up – it sounded gross, but I was pretty sure that wouldn't happen to me, since I was young and only had a hundred-plus pounds to lose, instead of three hundred. Besides, anything was better than being obese, even having flappy, old-people skin.

We already knew from the *New Yorker* article that we could expect to lose most of our excess weight in the first year after the operation, and I for one was eager to finish with the information sessions and make with the skinny, already! But the doctors wanted to be certain that we were fully informed about all the risks and complications, as well as all the ways our lives would change after the surgery. We'd sat in what felt like a hundred different-but-same neutrally decorated rooms, always in a semicircle with other aspiring patients. We listened to slender nurses, many of them newly thin, former patients themselves, list their favourite post-GB 'treats' and caution against the pitfalls of indulging. We were told that some people are so attached to food that they have a severe mental breakdown after the surgery, and sometimes they even have to have it reversed. We were counselled and told and warned and cautioned about all these changes the GB would bring, and we were given advice on how to handle them.

But what we weren't told was how much the GB might *not* change about our lives, and how to handle the disappointment that some of us might suffer when our worlds *weren't* flipped upside down. When my stomach hurt or my eyes watered from throwing up, I felt justified in soothing myself with images of my future self: slim and confident, even sexy, with curves in all the right places, no extra rolls or creases. I was convinced my life would change 180 degrees if I could just get through the recovery and lose enough weight.

Physically, the surgery was no walk in the park, but I expected that, and I could handle it. The answers all seemed pretty straightforward; we got personal trainers to hold us accountable at the gym; we ate mostly protein, when we could chew it well enough to keep it down; we started buying bottled water in bulk at Costco to encourage ourselves to drink more. We followed the rules, and the physical recovery went as smoothly as could be expected.

But I was wrong to think that everything would change so easily, or that my physical state was the only thing I needed to worry about. It wasn't just our bodies that had to recover and adapt to changes; there was an emotional journey ahead of us too. And despite all our information sessions and all my therapy appointments, I wasn't prepared for that process to be so difficult, and so goddamn *long*.

6

San Francisco, June 2002

'Oh my God, these would be *perfect* for Australia!' Andrea holds up a pair of boardshorts, or what pass for boardshorts in the women's section of PacSun. They're about the size of a sandwich, blue, with yellow stripes down the sides and a Velcro fly about two inches long. I paste an excited look over the prudish shock I feel creeping onto my face.

'Well, try them on, then!'

Andrea lets out a small squeak of excitement and dashes off to the dressing room. I turn to Courtney and allow the prudeface to return. She laughs.

'Yeah, well, you know Pea. She likes it short!'

I smile, relaxed by Courtney's presence on this shopping trip. Among the three of us, we cover a lot of body types. Andrea, who was the last of us to turn seventeen, has grown up to look pretty similar to the thirteen-year-old I first met: tall, straight, with a round booty and firm, muscular legs, helped along by her constant soccer and volleyball practices. Courtney and I, who met when we were both ten, have filled out very differently: she hasn't grown much in height, stopping at five foot three, but her body has morphed into a buxom hourglass with a small waist and curvy hips, and I've grown to be almost as tall as Andrea, but my width grew to surpass both girls put together. Now, six months after the GB and weighing in at around two hundred pounds, I'm small-waisted, bottom-heavy, and confused, unsure whether I'll lose more weight or level out, unsure whether I'm 'normal' yet or ever will be.

I reach past Courtney to the rack behind her and grab a strappy little sundress, white with multicoloured polka dots. I hold it against my foreign body and try to figure out whether it would fit. I haven't worked up the courage to try anything on yet today, even though the whole point of this shopping trip was for me to buy some new things to wear when Andrea and I go to Australia with her mom in July. I'm excited to be able to fly without the fear that the seatbelt won't close, but I'm terrified of two weeks of beaches and hot guys (if Heath Ledger, Andrea's and my recent obsession, is anything to go by). I'm especially nervous about the hot guys – despite losing so much weight, I'm still stuck on the Island of the Unfuckables, and I'm starting to wonder whether the weight is all that's keeping me there. Maybe there's something inherently unattractive about me ... *or maybe I just haven't lost enough weight.* I can only hope I'll keep getting smaller, and my skin will eventually tighten up.

For now, I still need new clothes. I put the sundress back and pick up a pair of shorts. I check the tag and a quiet scoff escapes from my throat. *Large? HA. They'd maybe fit my upper arms.* I put the shorts back and turn to Courtney.

'I don't know,' I muse, 'I guess if I had legs like Andrea's I'd probably wear all kinds of short-shorts and tight jeans too. Especially if I rocked a booty like that instead of this flat, wide ass I'm carrying around.' I stuff the shorts back into the rack.

Courtney nods. 'I think we're all a little jealous of that ass – God knows I'd like some more roundness in the back.' She shrugs, and her eyes scan the store. '*Ooh*, I really need a new one-piece.'

She heads over to the swimsuit section, but I hang back. I slide my right hand around behind myself, over the velvety corduroy that covers the flat, wide, jiggly shelf where my ass should be. I grab a handful of fat and pull it up, imagining what my back end would look like if I got butt implants like the ones J-Lo has made so popular. *Maybe that's what I need to balance out this shapeless beast of a body. Butt implants. And boobs, too.*

I glance down at my diminished chest. Where once my breasts spilled out of my 36C bra, now they just settle in the cups like exhausted puppies, the right one leaving a bit of a space between flesh and black lace, the left one overstepping its bounds just slightly. I reach into my top and adjust them to look more even, then follow Courtney, sidling through racks of clothes – even after losing the weight, I always move through aisles sideways, afraid if I walk straight I'll knock into them with my massive hips. When I reach her, she's holding up a low-cut brown halter suit with a ring between the breasts. I smile.

'Cute! Do you need a suit for something specific, or just to add to your wardrobe?'

'Eh, you know, sort of a "just in case" suit. I mean, my family might go on a trip or something this summer, the parents still haven't decided, but my old black one is really boring and it's starting to do that thing at the belly, you know?'

I nod – I know. 'Where it goes all sheer and nubbly.'

'Exactly! Ugh, why does it *do* that?'

'When I was a kid I always thought it was because of scraping the fabric against the pool edge when I pushed myself out, but now . . . I dunno.' I shrug and reach up to brush a wisp of hair behind my ear. *That was a mistake* – I'm disappointed all over again at how little of it there is. Losing so much weight so fast has meant that my best feature, my thick, wavy brown hair, has been diminished too, by about half. I turn toward the large mirror mounted by the fitting rooms, about twenty feet away, and try to check myself out subtly, keeping my eyes above the neck and pushing my thinning hair around to make sure I don't have any bald spots. Just as I'm starting to obsess a bit too much, Andrea's arm sticks out from behind one of the fitting-room doors and begins to wave.

'Hey, guys!' Andrea is beckoning to us. We make our way over there and she opens the door wider so we can see her clearly. She's wearing the shorts with no top, just her bra, because she wore a dress to come shopping and doesn't have anything to try them on with.

'Cute bra! I want one.' *I really need new bras. And new everything else, ugh.*

'Thanks! What do you think of the shorts? Too short? Do my thighs look fat?' She turns around to give us the back view. They're certainly short. I go first.

'Dude. They're super-short, I'm not gonna lie. But you definitely rock them like whoa – your ass looks *hot*. Hot stuff!'

I say this last part in the voice of Ross, from the TV show *Friends*. It's one of our favourite things to say – we often shout it at boys out of car windows: a drive-by hot-stuffing, we call it.

'Really?' Andrea turns anxiously to Courtney, and I hold my breath. Courtney's not one to lie, which is one reason I like shopping with her, but she can be a bit ... well, 'subtle as a brick to the face' is how I like to describe her. I think Andrea looks hot, if a *teeny bit* inappropriate, but that might just be the effect of wearing them without a shirt. And I also think she loves the shorts, which is the most important thing. *Anyway, she'll be wearing them on the beach or river rafting or something, and they're more modest than a bikini!*

But I'm not sure Courtney will see it the same way. She looks Andrea in the eye and gives her honest opinion.

'Well, they're way shorter than anything *I* would ever wear, but if you like them you should get them. There'll always be people wearing less than you, I'm sure!'

Andrea does her little happy dance – throwing her body from side to side and bouncing off the balls of her feet while making a goofy smiley face – and goes back into the dressing room to change. I look at Courtney.

'Nicely put.'

'Well, she obviously loves them, and it's not like her ass was *hanging out*.' She smiles at me in a snarky way and we exchange a look that says *unlike so many girls we see walking around everywhere*. I laugh and my anxiety about clothes releases slightly – if there's anybody who can make me feel like less of a freak for weighing more than a hundred pounds and wearing knee-length skirts, it's Courtney. She's always carried her own quirky/classic sense of style with the sort of confidence that makes anything she puts on look fantastic; she'll show up at the movie theatre in jeans with red suspenders and a cartoon-printed T-shirt with a girly cardigan over it, and a wave of envy will flood my brain, even if that outfit on someone else would elicit a snort of derision on any other day. I've always admired the fashion risks she takes, but these days what I really wish I could emulate is her confidence. *I wonder what it would feel like to be so sure of myself.* I turn to ask her, but she's wandered off toward the wall of sunglasses, and is now contemplating a pair of bright yellow square frames. I smile and head back to flip through the sale rack while we wait for Andrea.

Once Andrea has paid for the shorts, we get out of the bright colours and cheap fabrics that fill PacSun and head upstairs. Courtney wants to check out Banana Republic; we'll all need nice clothes soon for college interviews, and since none of us has ever had a real job (doing well in school was always my real job, Courtney has her art, and Andrea plays too many sports to have time for working as well as getting As) it's not like our closets are exactly overflowing with sensible skirt suits and tailored trousers. As the escalator bears us upwards along the edge of the open core of the mall, the smell of Mrs Fields' Cookies wafts up with us, and my stomach pinches. It's been so long since I've eaten something sweet that I almost don't remember what a chocolate-chip cookie tastes like – I haven't touched sugary stuff since the surgery, too afraid of the consequences. It feels weird, and kind of good, to resist my cravings – the same way it always felt, but better because it's lasted longer and I have more faith in its staying power this time. There's a Hundred Grand, a chocolate and caramel candy bar, sitting in the top drawer of my bedside table at home right now, and every evening I think about taking a tiny nibble but I always close the drawer with a nervous sigh. Now I feel wistful for a second, my mouth filling with saliva at the thought of a warm, gooey, soft cookie, but then I look up and see all the stores on the four floors above, and I remind myself why I'm here. To shop at *normal stores.*

At Banana Republic, I drift through the racks, letting my fingers skim the silks and cottons, touching everything before I even look at it. My hands trail over soft, thin cotton tees and slippery satin dresses; my eyes barely register each piece of clothing, noting only a strapless top here, a clingy skirt there. Everything I touch is more a wish than a possibility, even now. *Besides*, I think, *Banana is kind of spendy if you're just going to lose more weight and not fit into things again.* I can only hope I'll lose more weight. I'd sort of hoped to be skinny by now, even though the doctors said it would probably take a year to lose it all – I'm antsy to finish the conversion process and start my new life as a normal person.

My hovering fingers pause at a heavy cotton material, and my eyes take their cue. The pants are black with a light grey pinstripe. The outer material is the heavy cotton I felt first, but upon inspection they prove to be lined with something satiny and black, probably polyester. Out of curiosity, I check the tag: 14. I sigh and move to put the pants back – I'm a 16–18 on the bottom these days, last I checked – but Courtney has snuck up on me and grabs the hanger from me.

'Hey, these are nice! Are you going to try them on?'

I make a feeble attempt to take them back, but she either ignores me or doesn't notice. She's checking the tag for a size. I try to head her off at the pass.

'No, I don't think they'd fit. Too bad, 'cause I kinda like them and it's not like I have any pants to wear to interviews or graduation or whatever.'

'These will totally fit you!' Courtney is holding the waistband up against my hips. I move back, afraid she might accidentally touch me and feel the icky softness of my emptying body.

'No, they're a fourteen.'

'So? You never know with sizes, and anyway those pants you're wearing are falling off you, and what're they, a sixteen?'

'I dunno, eighteen?' The pants *are* hanging a little low in the crotch, but I figured that was just because they're men's, from the sports store where my brother likes to shop. I have no idea what size they would be in women's numbers.

'Look, just try them on. You haven't tried anything on all day. If you hate them, I won't make you try on anything else, and you can go to Australia naked for all I care.'

The thought of being anywhere naked makes me grab the pants like they're the last ass-shelf-covering on earth. I clutch them to me and head for the dressing room without another word, leaving Courtney grinning smugly after me.

The door clicks closed behind me and I breathe out. I look at my new face – high cheekbones, pointed chin, small, narrow nose – in the full-length mirror and whisper 'Here goes nothing,' then I turn my back to my watchful eyes and pull down my corduroys. I don't need to unbutton them, just work them down over my hips, catching my undies with a fingertip so they're not pulled off too. *I guess Courtney was right about these being a little big . . .*

I pick up the pants from the bench and unclip them from their hanger. *The moment of truth.* I hold my breath as I unzip them and step into the legs. Slowly, afraid to rip the seams, I lift the waistband up over my knees. *So far, so good.* I pull them higher, shocked at the way the lining slithers easily over the lumps and bumps of my thighs. I shiver, and my skin gets goosebumps. I take one more deep breath, suck in my stomach, and pull once more – the fabric slides easily over my butt and hips and there I am, clothed. No tears, no rips, no nervous breakdowns. Just me, in a pair of pants.

I button them and zip them up, and then I turn around to face myself.

I damn near cry when I see my reflection. *Oh my fucking God. I'm normal.* My body looks . . . like a normal body. Two legs, two arms. Hips, butt, boobs, a waist. That face. For the first time since the surgery, I look like a real person. All the body parts I've been inspecting and pushing and pulling have come together for one glorious moment and shown me a whole picture: a girl, almost a woman, who could very easily be headed for a college interview, or to work as an editor at my dream publishing house, or to school, where a class full of eager English students await my thoughts on their latest short stories. A normal girl, almost a woman, with a normal body (if a bit overweight and thick through the bottom half), and a normal life ahead of her.

I'm still staring at myself with my mouth open when Courtney bangs on the door and shouts, 'Woman! What are you *doing* in there? Show us the goods!'

I open the door and grin like an idiot as Courtney and Andrea gape at me.

'Oh my god, banana, you look so HOT!' Andrea looks positively gleeful.

'Well, I wouldn't go that far, but they're not bad, are they?' There's no way I feel hot, but I've waited so long to just feel normal that I'm practically spinning.

'No, Anne, I'd go that far. Those pants are definitely hot.' Courtney stares at my hips as she says this, then moves her eyes up to my waist. 'You look super curvaceous. Damn.'

I grin at her and don't even think about fighting the blush I know is coating my face.

'So that's a yes, then? I don't even know how much they cost yet!'

Both girls shake their heads, and Andrea says what we're all thinking.

'I haven't seen you smile like that in a dressing room ... *ever*. Get them.'

I shut the door and lean against it. I almost don't want to take the pants off. *What if I buy them and then when I get home it turns out I was wrong to think I looked good, and really I am this Raggedy-Ann doll made up of all these disgusting parts and it was just a momentary lapse of judgement?* I look in the mirror one more time. The pants fit perfectly.

Before I can change my mind, I whip them off, throw on my corduroys and shoes, and charge through the store, headed for the cash register and a $75 (on sale) confirmation of the normalcy I've chased for so many years.

*

Of course, within a month, my body had changed again and the pants didn't fit so perfectly any more. The waistband dug just a bit into the soft skin of my belly, the legs flapped a little in the empty inch of space around my thighs, and the butt sagged just enough to make my pancake ass look even flatter. But for three glorious weeks I was the proud owner of a pair of size 14 Banana Republic pinstriped pants, and those weeks of wear were worth every penny. For years, when shopping for pants was one of my worst nightmares and often ended with me in tears in a dressing room piled with mountains of discarded jeans, the memory of that one pair of beautiful, flattering trousers was enough to keep me going.

The more consistent shopping success started with, and continued to depend on, dresses. I'd always been bottom-heavy, and that didn't change after the surgery; as I gathered the courage to try on clothes at normal-sized stores for the first time in over five years, I quickly cottoned on to the fact that dresses were extremely forgiving. All a full-skirted dress had to fit was my ribcage, and then the fabric would work around the rest of me. And my ribcage, it turned out, was a pretty average size under all that fat. By the summer after the surgery my torso could fit into a size 12 dress, and sometimes even a 10! I was in heaven. I bought dress after dress: Banana Republic, the Gap, even one from Anthropologie's sale rack. But the truest thrill was fitting into that one pair of pants.

Even after I lost the majority of the weight, my lower body was still pretty hefty: in jeans or pants I was a good two sizes larger than I was in dresses or tops. Which meant, at the time, a size 18, sometimes 16 on a thin day — most American stores only carry up to a size 14, if you're lucky, a 12 or even a 10 if you're not. So for a long time I was still wearing my internet catalogue jeans and my men's corduroys on days when it was too cold to wear my pretty cotton dresses or jersey skirts. I avoided shopping for new jeans at all costs; trying on pants was enough to make me dissolve into tears in a way that ill-fitting dresses didn't. With dresses, I could convince myself that the garment in question was simply too small, or weirdly cut, but with pants the fault was always mine: my flat, wide ass, my thick, squishy thighs, my gross, overhanging stomach.

And all those villainous body parts were indeed to blame, not just for too-tight pant legs or gapping waistbands, but for everything that was still wrong in my life, even after I'd lost a hundred pounds. Sure, I was doing well in school, especially in English and Spanish, and I had plans to go to college and get a job where I could use my love of writing and reading to pay the rent. I had a great group of friends who made me feel like the funny, thoughtful, clever girl I had decided was really there inside the layers of self-consciousness – she peeked out sometimes when I was really comfortable with my surroundings, and she could even be quite brazen under the right circumstances. But I would have to make myself comfortable with my permanent surroundings – my body – if I wanted to convince her to come out more often, and eventually stay visible permanently.

I was working on it. It took just under a year for the majority of the excess weight to drop off. I went on an exchange programme to Spain about four weeks after the surgery, and my new clothes were hanging off me by the end of the trip. I threw up a lot of paella in those two weeks in Valencia, but I was still fat, a fact of which the Spanish weren't shy of reminding me. One day I went to the beach with my friend's host family, and the mother ordered me into the middle of the back seat, turned to my friend with a warm smile on her face, and said: 'She's a big girl, no?' During the school week, I got a lot of stares on campus, and once a boy leaned his head out the window when I was in the courtyard and started shouting 'McDonald's, McDonald's,' over and over, in my direction. I found it a bit ironic that this trip, when I was smaller than I'd been in years, was the first time I'd really ever been bullied by strangers about my weight, but for once in my life I wasn't devastated by the comments – I was beginning to see more of the girl my friends liked so much, and I was still losing. Whenever I felt uncomfortable about my size or self-conscious in front of boys, I just distracted my nervous mind with images of the body I was sure awaited me on the other side: sleek, slim, and smooth. My hips would be round, like Marilyn Monroe's, instead of lumpy and wide; my waist would be tiny, sloping up and out to a full, proportional bust; my legs would look longer and straighter. I was sure I'd be skinny and beautiful before that stupid bully even made it to second base with a girl.

By the time my junior year ended, in June, I was probably down about ninety pounds. I felt like I'd lost most of it from my face (and my boobs, *damnit*), but the rest of me was shrinking too. I was starting to get excited about how thin I'd be. The clothes I'd wear. The boys who would suddenly want to date me. And I kept on losing. When I dropped below the two hundred mark, though, it slowed down. I wasn't shedding more than a pound or two per week, while my dad, who had already lost a larger percentage of his original weight than I had and was even beginning to look a bit gaunt, was still dropping; he wouldn't stop raving about how his pants didn't fit, and I could barely stand to be in a room with him. The doctors had warned us about the tapering off, but I didn't understand why I was plateauing while my dad was still getting slimmer, and it scared the crap out of me. And for good reason – by August I'd stopped losing weight, at 185 pounds. Still way too high if you asked me (or any women's magazine).

For once in my life, I was doing everything right: I was taking my vitamins, eating almost exclusively protein at meals, not snacking, exercising with a personal trainer. I hadn't touched a candy bar or cookie since going under the knife (I was way too terrified of dumping!), and I was even starting to like veggies and salad almost as much as I liked meat and carbs. It was kind of weird to find myself craving asparagus or grilled zucchini, but it felt great to be able to express my desire for a big, crunchy salad and not feel like a total fraud. My dad, on the other hand, was dumping regularly and still eating too fast at meals, which meant throwing up afterwards. I couldn't understand why *I* was the one who'd hit a wall – why was I being punished for good behaviour? I also didn't understand why my body didn't look the way I'd pictured it. During the recovery, when I'd occupied my drug-addled mind with fantasy images of myself, I'd imagined myself svelte and beautiful. Lithe. Taut. I'd expected my dad to be a little saggy – he was old when he lost the weight – but I'd been told, and I'd believed it, that because I was so young my skin was more likely to bounce back, especially if I exercised regularly. Realistically, I expected to look like a normal teenager, maybe not as sleek as my fantasies, but with legs and arms and a stomach that were firm, at least.

I was anything *but* firm. I was a freak. Inhuman. Like

nothing I'd ever seen before, on real people or in magazines or TV. And that's where my obsession with my reflection started: in an attempt to figure out what I really looked like.

Sometimes I would stand in front of my bathroom mirror for fifteen minutes, just pushing and pulling my skin this way and that. My stomach hung down, emptied of most of the fat that once held it out from my skeleton, and I would grab great handfuls of it and lift, then drop: *skinny, fat, skinny, fat.* I stared at my body from every angle, trying to see what others saw. I stared at other women too, on the street, in the airport, at the supermarket, sizing them up, slotting myself in where I thought I fit: *Am I fatter than she is? Or skinnier? Or the same size, but with bigger hips and smaller boobs?*

I spent hours looking at plastic-surgery websites, comparing before and after photos and trying to imagine my body in the same way. I segmented myself: hips, thighs, boobs, butt, waist, knees, arms. I was a rag doll, a bunch of body parts stitched together at awkward angles, no one part really fitting with another. I could only see myself in pieces; when I tried to pull back and look at the whole picture the image blurred and I had to close my eyes to keep from getting dizzy. So I focused on the bits, doing squats and biceps curls to try to 'fix' my thighs and upper arms, buying pair after pair of big granny panties to cover my hanging stomach, hoping that my skin might bounce back suddenly and spare me the awkward conversation with my parents wherein I would have to admit that I wanted even more surgery. While I waited for my body to fix itself, trying to hold out hope that my skin was just in shock and would eventually recover, I searched out clothes that hid my problem areas, knee-length dresses that flowed over my jiggling hips and skimmed my knock knees, short little cardigans to hide my massive bingo wings, padded bras to perk up my sagging, uneven breasts. Little fixes for each section of the whole.

This compartmentalising of my body made clothes shopping a nightmare. The minute I tried something on and looked in the mirror I would zero in on sections of myself: *Does it make my hips look too saddlebaggy? My boobs too droopy? My butt too flat?* I was completely unable to see the overall picture, and I couldn't even begin to answer the question: *How does this look on me?*

Oddly enough, this was a downturn from my shopping attitude when I was fat. Back then, I was so riddled with 'problem areas' that my whole body became one big problem, which meant that I was happy just to have articles of clothing zip or button, and if they looked nice I was ecstatic. When I lost the weight, though, my expectations changed. It was no longer enough just to be clothed and remotely decent-looking, now I wanted to look good. And God *forbid* any excess skin hang out or droop over a waistband. I must have been a nightmare to shop with.

Luckily, my friends hung in there. They trudged through shopping malls with me, gave me honest feedback on the few items I had the courage to try on, and propped me up with coffee and chatter when something didn't fit. My friends had made life worth living when I was fat and ready to throw in the towel, and now they were a constant reminder that just because my body didn't change completely right away, that didn't mean I shouldn't keep trying to find a style that suited it. And that funny, clever girl they all liked so much, the reason they shopped with me and soothed my ragged self-esteem? She started to appear more and more, despite my continued discomfort with the body she was trapped in. It turned out, even if I hadn't fixed my self-image issues yet, the simple knowledge that I wasn't alone in my struggle was enough to make me that little bit more comfortable in my saggy skin.

7

St Louis, Missouri, May 2004

I'm in my dorm room, staring at the phone and willing myself to text him, when he knocks on the open door. Somehow I know it's him before I even turn around, and my chest tightens. I swivel in the chair and pretend to be pleased to see him.

'Wesley! Hey! What are you doing here?'

'I came to see if you wanted to grab lunch at the cafeteria.'

His voice is deep and a little husky, matching his appearance perfectly. Wes looks like he's just stepped out of a classier time, with a Clark Gable-y bone structure, casually perfect hair, and a tall, broad-shouldered body that's ideal for his slightly vintage, hipster style of dress. He's gorgeous, but unfortunately he knows it.

'Lunch? Yeah, sure.' I try to act casual, as if I were just hanging out doing homework when he happened by, instead of lecturing myself about what I have to tell him. *But what do I have to tell him? That I think he's hot? That'll just feed his ego, and besides, it's not the point.*

I grab my ID card and keys and slip on my flip-flops and

we head for the student centre. My sandals crack like gun-shots on the cement stairs. The sound echoes around us and relieves me of the need to talk. Outside, though, there's no safety net. The air is still, warm. The large grass 'Swamp' that the dorm buildings surround is normally packed with stu-dents, but today it's deserted. The weather is getting hot and humid; the stifling St Louis summer will be upon us soon, but the good news is I'll be headed back to San Francisco by the time it gets really bad. Three months of old friends, fam-ily time, and best of all no boy drama – at least if he rejects me I don't have to see him until September.

'You OK?' Wes looks at me funny, cocking his head to the side and squinting, as if to convey that he is in fact capable of caring about the answer to his question. I feel my chest squish up into itself again, and I try to remember that I mean less to him than he'd have me believe. *Although I am one of his best friends, or I think I am . . .*

'Yeah, no, I mean . . .'

He raises his eyebrows and I try to laugh.

'Well, I have something to talk to you about, but it can wait until we sit down.'

Jesus, Anne, cryptic much? Why do you have to make things even more awkward than they already are? I shoot him a lighthearted, 'No-worries-it's-nothing-I'm-just-weird' smile. He smiles back, a little warily, and changes the subject.

'Hey, what did you think of those Radiohead CDs I loaned you? Pretty awesome, huh?'

I remember the two CDs I burned onto my computer,

live recordings of some of Radiohead's more obscure per-
formances. I haven't even listened to them yet.

'Oh, yeah, totally awesome.' I say what I know he really
wants to hear: 'Where did you even get them? I mean, I've
never even heard of any of those songs before!'

Wes beams with pride and I mentally pat myself on the
back. *Yup, nothing like stroking the old music ego to make a
boy feel special. Even a nineteen-year-old virgin knows that
much.*

'Yeah, no, they're like totally underground. You know
they only played those songs at one concert, in England four
years ago, and there are only, like, ten recordings in the US.
So yeah, they're pretty hard to find.'

'Yeah, thanks for loaning them to me.'

We walk quietly for a bit, sticking alongside the looming
cement-block dorm buildings for shade, the dry grass
crunching under our feet. I revel in the peace of his comfort
with me, making sure to drink in every drop before I ruin
it for ever. I think about the winter formal last month, to
which we both showed up with different groups of friends,
neither of us with a date.

I wore my senior prom dress, a beautiful strapless number,
dusky rose satin covered in swiss-dot black lace, in a flattering fifties shape – I'd bought it at BCBG, a normal store for
normal-sized girls, and I loved it for what it represented *and*
how it made me look: curvy, slim-waisted, and womanly. On
my feet were my favourite pumps: also a soft, dark rose colour, with a white leather trim and little white leather flowers

on the outside edge. A white leather heel, too, about five inches high. They were excruciating.

But the pain was worth it when I saw Wes, in his forties sportscoat and trousers, with black-and-white saddle shoes that seemed the soul mates of my beautiful pumps. We took a picture of our feet side by side, nearly nuzzling. Bliss. He paid more attention to me that night than ever before, dancing with me and complimenting me; I could even swear I'd seen a glint of jealousy in his eyes when I danced close to my friend Mark, with Joe man-wiching me from the other side. That was the night I decided that it might not be the end of the world to let myself believe what all my friends had been insisting: he seemed to be into me too.

But it's been a while since then, and I haven't heard much from him. Until he showed up at my door today, in fact, I hadn't seen him in weeks. We've all been busy with end-of-term papers and exams, so I brushed it off, but I can't help feeling like he would have called if that night had meant as much to him as it did to me.

I shake the negative thoughts out of my head, trying to replace them with my knowledge of boys' timidity and laziness. Wes holds the door for me as we walk into the blast of air conditioning that fills the main building. We greet fellow floor-mates and classmates as we walk through the hall to the cafeteria, and I try not to feel like they're all staring at us, wondering what on earth I could possibly bring to this relationship. *They probably think I do his homework for him. Which I probably would.*

I take my time deciding what to eat, stalling as long as

I can. I've promised Andrea I'll do it today, in person, and the sooner I get it over with the longer I'll have to hide in my room and cry afterwards. But that doesn't mean I'm raring to go. While Wes is ordering something high-calorie and delicious at the grill, I hover at the salad station, trying to convince my churning stomach to find something tempting, and something that won't make it churn louder and embarrass me further. Finally, because the guy behind the counter is waiting for me, I request a small chopped mozzarella salad with oil and vinegar instead of a pre-mixed dressing. The vinegar is balsamic, a dark, dangerous colour, and I flash forward to an image of my chin, dribbling thick black liquid onto my chest. I shake the vision out of my mind, grab my salad, and head for the cashier, ignoring the huge Rice Krispies Treats and sugar cookies piled up next to the line.

I swipe my card to pay for my lunch and Wes's; he's out of points for the year, so I've offered to take him out for meals any time. *Oh, God, that's probably why he wanted to go to lunch with me! I'm such an idiot.* I force myself to smile at the lady as she hands back my card, and try not to pass out as Wes puts a gentle hand on my back and steers me toward a table by the window. *OK, OK, maybe that's not the only reason. Remember what the girls always say: he wouldn't seek you out if he didn't enjoy your company, and he wouldn't have said you looked gorgeous at the formal if he didn't mean it. Boys don't just say shit like that. It has to at least mean he loves you as a friend, and if that's true then he won't think you're ridiculous for even thinking he might feel something more . . . Worth a shot. That's what they said. It's worth a shot.*

Wes is staring at me like I'm crazy, and I realise I've been taking deep, yoga-y breaths to try to keep from throwing up or crying. I haven't felt this emotionally uncontrolled since high school, not that high school was so long ago. I laugh awkwardly.

'Ugh, sorry, it's just the trees blooming, setting off my asthma a little . . . no biggie.'

Wes makes a face that suggests concern, again, then his eyes open wide and he looks down at his plate.

'Sssht! Don't turn around,' he hisses. I'm already half turned in my seat, trying to see what's given him such a fright, and to play it off I pretend I'm just cracking my back. I twist the other way, keeping up the charade, then I face him.

'What is it?'

'Rosie.' He makes a pained face. Rosie is Wes's ex-girlfriend, a quiet, clever Hispanic girl with perfect slim curves and a lightly freckled, gently beautiful face. She broke up with him a month ago, after rumours spread that he'd done drugs and had a threesome in a hot tub with a young married couple in town. I never had the courage to ask him if it was true.

'Oh. Well you should go say hi . . .' I wonder if he believes my casual tone. I've spent far too much time helping him try to win her back in recent weeks, buying her favourite candy at the grocery store so he can give it to her, listening to him spout empty, clichéd comments about how much he still likes her, giving out advice like Dear Abby, pretending I want him to be happy.

I don't want him to be happy. I want him to be miserable. *Then maybe I'll start to look like a viable option – better than nothing, at least?*

'No way. She's with that asshole.'

I turn, no longer caring if they see me. Wes hisses again, but I ignore him. Rosie's new boyfriend is tall, skinny, nerdy-looking in that floppy-haired, reads-philosophy, listens-to-Chopin kind of way. Clever-looking. They seem happy together. Wes hates him.

I force down a bite of my salad. Wes has already eaten half his sandwich, but at the sight of Rosie he's set it down with a disgusted look on his handsome face. He hasn't touched it since.

My phone rings and I pull it out of my pocket. It's Andrea. I'm not sure why she'd be calling, since she knows I'm supposed to be confessing my feelings to Wes, but I answer it, glad for further stalling that doesn't involve girls who are prettier and thinner than I am.

'Hey! What's up?'

'Banana, I had a thought. I don't want you to tell him you like him.'

'What?' I smile at Wes and mouth *Sorry* at him. He's still staring at Rosie.

'I mean, I think you should ask him out instead!' Andrea has just read a book about how rejection is a good thing because it frees you up to find the right person, and now she's on an honesty kick.

'Andrea,' now it's my turn to hiss. I turn my head away from Wes, hoping he won't hear. Or maybe hoping he'll hear just enough to relieve me of having to say it. 'I'm not even sure I can do *this*, much less that.'

'I'm just saying, then he'd know, but it wouldn't just be leaving the confession out there in the open for *him* to do something with! You'd kill two birds with one stone!'

I wish I felt half as excited as she sounds. Instead I feel the little bit of mozzarella I've managed to eat hovering at the base of my throat, threatening to come back up. I swallow, hard.

'Look, I can't talk about this right now. I'll call you later, OK?'

'You better! I want to hear all about your date!'

I sigh. Andrea has so much faith that boys will eventually realise that I'm not hideous. *I wish I believed her.*

I close the phone and glance up at Wes.

'Sorry about that. Just Andrea.'

I take a deep breath, as deep as I can get it without coughing, and then I say it.

'Wes, I told you I had to tell you something . . .'

Wes puts his hand up to stop me. He's been watching me intently ever since I turned my face away and lowered my voice on the phone.

'I think I know what it is.'

'You do?' I'm relieved I don't have to say it out loud, but the expression on his face tells me I don't want to hear what's coming next.

'Yeah, and I just, well, I don't . . .'

'Yeah, no. Totally cool. This never happened.' It's my turn to cut him off and spare him the awkward words. 'We're just having lunch. Nothing happened that was out of the ordinary.'

I can feel my face burning, but I try to pretend I don't notice. I take a huge bite of salad and stuff it in my mouth like a frat boy, as if to prove that I don't have a wounded female heart. *See? No biggie! Just havin' lunch with my bro!*

Wes smiles. It's fake, but it'll do.

'So, you excited to get home for the summer?'

I nod probably too vigorously, still chewing, and give him the thumbs up. He laughs a little, relaxes. I pretend to relax too.

It's over. It's over, I did it (sort of), and it wasn't so bad. We're still friends.

I know I'm lying to myself, but I can deal with the mortification and tears and self-loathing when I'm alone. For now, I just chew and smile, chew and smile.

*

Even after I lost a hundred pounds, even when I could fit into the same clothes as some of my friends, even when my face appeared, pointy-chinned and high-cheekboned, from the fat, I still felt completely invisible to boys.

Some small part of me had hoped that when I lost the weight, boys would sit up and notice. Like Audrey Hepburn in *Sabrina* – I'd just cut my hair and drop a few dress sizes and suddenly I'd be the belle of the ball, someone fresh in a sea of old news. Ha.

When I got back to high school after my surgery, I was still fat. Never mind that I lost thirty pounds in the first two weeks; it took a while to lose enough weight for people to notice. And they did notice, the following fall, when I showed up 110 pounds lighter for my senior year. They noticed, and they complimented me on how good I looked, but it was kind of like I'd shown up with a well-suited Mohawk: I was a pleasant shock, rather than an object of desire. *Hey, the fatty's not so fat any more! Cool!*

I told myself that college would be different. These high-school boys knew what I had been, and they couldn't see past it. That's what I told myself. *College will be different. Clean slate, new boys, no fat-girl past.* Besides, I was going to a university in the middle of the country, leaving city life, where everybody is a vegan and has a gym membership and worries about losing five pounds, for a more authentic place, where men liked *real* women. I made it through my senior year of high school by riding on that wave of hope about college – it allowed me to focus on passing the International Baccalaureate and getting into a good school and spending time having fun with the friends I'd be leaving soon, instead of wallowing all the time in my loneliness and my disappointment with the non-effect the surgery had had on my love life.

This isn't to say that the weight loss had *no* effect on my attitude about guys in high school, but it had more of an effect when I was outside school grounds. I no longer felt like the inappropriate attention from skeezers was somehow my punishment for being so disgusting that nobody else would come close. I got a bit better at giving contemptuous looks and moving away from roaming hands, and I even started to believe that maybe the random guy staring at me from across the street thought I was cute, rather than immediately assuming my dress was caught in my underwear or I had chocolate smeared all over my face. I wasn't *always* a joke any more.

But at the same time, I began to occupy a strange limbo: I wasn't fat enough to be the object of somebody's fantasy or fetish, but I wasn't thin enough to be a 'hottie' in the usual socially accepted way. In certain situations, I felt even more invisible than before, relegated even deeper into the Island of the Unfuckables; I didn't elicit extreme disgust, but I also had less chance of eliciting extreme excitement. I wasn't sure how to feel about that, given that I never wanted to be anyone's fetish ... but better a fetish than too boring to glance at twice, right?

When I got to college, I had been 'thinnish' for over a year. I had been to Australia with Andrea, and we had flirted shamelessly with a shop assistant in Double Bay. I had gone to my senior prom with friends, and even let myself believe that I might have a chance to hook up with a cute Russian boy we met in the hotel lobby – and when another girl got there first, I'd almost managed to convince myself that it was timing and courage I lacked, not looks. I had spent the summer after high school travelling with Andrea and Courtney through western Europe, flirting with Italian men, wearing dresses half the size of my previous wardrobe, and even going topless at a secluded nudist beach in France (Courtney started it, and Andrea and I followed suit, giggling the whole time and covering our nipples). I was slowly beginning to think that maybe things *were* different; maybe I *was* someone that people might find attractive. Sure, I still felt obese a lot of the time (on the plane to Paris I'd walked sideways down the aisle and winced any time I brushed against someone, and I refused to sit down on the Métro unless there were three seats available – one for me and one for each hip) and I was still a bigger size than all of my friends, but at least I could shop at the same stores as the girls, and as disgusting as *I* thought my excess skin was, I tried to convince myself that it wasn't noticeable to other people. College was to be my last test of the theory that I wasn't gross, I just thought I was – if other people found me attractive, people who didn't know my history with weight troubles, then maybe I could find a way to believe that the repulsive person I saw in the mirror was really all in my head.

So I sucked it up, and sucked it in, and gave mixed-gender social interaction another try. My freshman floor was co-ed, so there were guys around all the time; there was even a room at the end of the hall where the guys had what we girls dubbed 'naked time'. There were three of them, one skinny Catholic kid and two *extremely* well-formed basketball players. One was beautiful and smart and funny, and the other was six feet eight inches tall – enough said. These guys used to sit around shirtless, reading and studying and just generally airing out their nipples. College was the best thing I'd ever done.

But these guys weren't accessible to me. Well, the skinny one probably was, given that he used to come to my room and sketchily snuggle up on me and tell me how girls were so mean while looking intensely into my eyes. But for once

I wasn't interested in the attainable. If I was going to prove to myself that I was finally attractive, I wanted to appeal to a guy that I also found attractive. I didn't need a six-foot-eight basketball player or a sexy rock star in a band or even a super-cool hipster dude – I just wanted someone who was interesting for his own merits, rather than being attractive solely for his acceptance of my looks.

And then Wes came along. I'd met him the previous summer at orientation weekend, but it wasn't anything more than a drooling-over-his-face kind of attraction until he remembered me that fall and sought out my friendship. I, of course, was fully prepared to avoid him and pretend I didn't remember him, because I'd rather be kind of a bitch than have people think of me as 'that pathetic fatty who fell all over me'. But then he went and wanted to be friends. And I fell hard. Really hard.

It was just like high school: any indication that he liked me and I swooned. He'd cross the quad to say hello in front of friends, and I'd blush fiercely and make fun of him to deflect attention from my obvious affection; he'd come by my room to ask a quick question about the cooking club I was in, and I'd drop everything to find out the answer; he'd send me a text to let me know he was going to a party and ask if I was going to be there, and I'd scramble to get someone to play wing woman and throw together a cute outfit.

Wes was different from my high-school crushes in one very important regard, though: he was good-looking. Like, really really ridiculously good-looking. And for the first time in my life that was all that mattered to me. I didn't care that he was arrogant, or that we had little in common besides our mutual affection for his looks. I didn't care that he only showed up to hang out when he needed something, or that he checked out other girls when we were together. He was *just so pretty.*

I was ashamed of my shallow feelings for Wes, but no amount of shame or self-reproach could stop them from growing into a crush of monstrous proportions. So even though it was miserably embarrassing, I was glad he rejected me at the end of that first year, because if I hadn't had the balls to tell him I liked him, and he hadn't had the balls to say 'No way, José,' I probably would have swooned over him all through college. And that would have been way more humiliating than any rejection.

Besides, Wes's disinterest freed me up to see the other boys who existed in the world, and amazingly I did meet a guy the following year. There I was, minding my own business and enjoying the unseasonably warm early March weather at a little park near campus, and a cute guy came up to me and started a conversation. And then, shock of shocks, he asked me if I wanted to go out some time! I walked back to campus in a haze of disbelief; I had a real date.

His name was Josiah, an old-school biblical name on a modern American boy, which was a contrast I found really sexy. Also adorable were his slightly crooked smile and dark hair, just long enough to flop over his eyes a bit. His height was a little less of a draw: he wasn't much taller than I was, and on that first date (which *actually happened*), when I wore low heels, I felt like a giant.

But I also felt, for the first time in my life, like a normal girl. *So this is what first dates are like*, I kept thinking as I sipped my huge mug of tea and crossed my legs under the table, subtly adjusting the waistband on my jeans to hide the soft skin of my belly. We made small talk – families, friends, his ex, his dog – and drank our hot beverages in the tiny cafe with framed deco posters on the walls. I sneaked looks now and then at the other patrons, trying to catch them staring at this weird pair, the cute guy and the fatty, but they were all busy with their laptops and books. Nobody seemed to notice how freakish it was that I was on a date.

And then he took me home, in his old blue pickup truck (a stick shift – *swoon*), and walked me to my dorm door. And my heart felt like it was going to beat straight out of my chest and into his face as he leaned in to kiss me, and ... *I dodged the wrong way*. I totally fucked it up. He ended up making it into an awkward hug, and I fled into my suite and fell on the common-room floor, writhing in awkwardness and trying not to cry as I told my roommates how I'd screwed up my first kiss at the age of twenty. Our common-room window looked out on the street where Josiah had parked, so my roommates, concerned girlfriends that they were, dragged my squirming body out of view and tucked it into my room, then spent the next hour trying to convince me that I hadn't ruined everything.

Amazingly, I hadn't. I emailed him to say I'd had a nice time, and he emailed back asking me on another date. I couldn't believe I'd gotten another chance, and when he came to pick me up, to take me to the botanical gardens (in the freezing dead of late winter), I walked out of my dorm, put my hands on his shoulders, and kissed him on the lips. 'There,' I said, 'now that that's out of the way ... shall we go?' It was a lot more awkward and less bold/sexy than I'd imagined it, but it did the trick. We must have stopped to make out about a hundred times during our tour of the barren, wintry gardens.

And from there I just ran with it. I'd been waiting years for a guy to want to kiss me, to want to *do stuff* with me, and I wasn't going to wait any longer. I was even antsy enough to forget for a second that my 190-pound body was too saggy to show anyone, or that I hadn't told him the history of the scars on my stomach – I didn't have time to worry about that stuff, and anyway the scars were only about an inch long, and only two of them were visible (the third was inside my belly button). I pushed straight through the fears and concerns that had occupied my mind for the past three years, and I invited him back to my place for coffee, which I made in my French press and which we drank quickly before disappearing to my room. And then, all of a sudden, I was sexually experienced. We still hadn't done *it*, but we'd done pretty much everything else, and when he left that evening my roommates gathered around me and congratulated me, teasing me mercilessly for my glowing face and telling me how they'd all put earphones in 'just in case'.

Things with Josiah weren't perfect. They weren't even normal, really. We mostly communicated via email, since that's how we'd first gotten in touch after meeting at the park (thank you, Facebook), which meant I could go days without hearing from him. Which was thoroughly annoying. In fact, after our third date, I didn't hear from him for a week, at which point I finally found my self-respect and sent him a terse, pissed-off email telling him to man up and let me know if he was no longer interested. He apologised profusely and took me out to dinner that very night. So I slept with him.

The first time I'd gotten naked in front of Josiah, after the botanical gardens, I'd been mortified; all the body hatred I'd ignored in my hurry to get him behind a locked door came rushing back the instant I was fully nude. I'd covered myself as best I could and wished only for more arms, to be an octopus so I could hide every roll and jiggle and slump. But I couldn't hide it all, and Josiah had seen me. And he hadn't run away. He'd looked at me, told me not to be self-conscious (*as if*), and continued hooking up with me. And as difficult as it was to allow myself to be distracted from my body, I'd eventually managed to let the thrill of sexual encounter take over.

But later, when we had sex, I looked up at his throat, his head angled up and away from me, his arms flexed beside my neck and his shoulders moving over mine, and realised something that made the intimacy even easier: as long as I was on the bottom, and we were face to face, *he couldn't see below my shoulders*. With the reassurance of bodily invisibility, I was surprisingly quick to learn how to enjoy sex in the moment, and worry about how I looked later. Sex was the first bodily experience I'd ever had that could make me forget to hate my body, even if it was just for five minutes. Suddenly my body was there solely to receive pleasure, rather than being a sort of shell that constantly projected my inadequacy and personal failings to the world.

I'd told myself I'd wait until we were exclusive, at least. We weren't. But I was under no illusions about waiting for love; I was twenty years old, for Christ's sake, and I just wanted to get rid of the VIRGIN stamp on my forehead while I had the chance. So once he wasn't annoying me, and because he had a condom in his wallet, I let him have my V-card. And I didn't regret it one bit. It wasn't the most transcendent 'first time' ever, but neither was it bad. I could even feel a stirring of some future pleasure behind the pain. And afterwards, positioned just so (extra hip tucked, arm over roll), lying on his chest on top of my purple jersey sheets, I felt ... different. Or, I should say, I no longer felt *so different*. I felt like a normal girl, with a normal, slightly unsatisfying sex life. *I had a sex life*.

From that moment forward, something changed about the way I viewed my body – it wasn't just about me, any more. All of a sudden, my self-image was inextricably linked to an outside source, a *real* love life, or at least a real potential. Whereas, before Josiah, my hideous form was just the first in line for theoretical blame when I felt permanently single, now there was another judge on the panel, and this one was real, even tangible; the simple fact that someone else had seen me naked and decided to have sex with me anyway meant the bitch in my head wasn't the only person who could have an opinion about how I looked. And, better yet, her opinion began to matter less when there was an opposing (male) voice in the room.

I was thrilled to have found Josiah. I had, if not a legitimate boyfriend, at least a boy I was dating. A guy who took me for drives in his pickup; put his cool, dry hand on my thigh when he wasn't shifting; watched me get naked and didn't lose his hard-on. A guy who kissed me in front of my roommates and held my hand when we walked along the main street by campus, who wasn't afraid to be seen with me in a romantic way (I used to wish we would run into Wes, but alas we never did).

But he was also a guy who didn't feel strongly enough about me to have sex with me more than twice – and who, after that second time, sat behind me on the floor of his bedroom (he'd just moved in and didn't have a bed yet), wrapped his arms around my naked body and played snippets of obscure songs from his laptop to impress me with his musical knowledge (this is known to have the opposite effect on me). A guy with whom I had little real connection; who didn't even bother to say goodbye to me before I went home for the summer; who may or may not have gone home with someone else just a week after he told me he wasn't sleeping with anyone but me.

In truth, he was just another guy: funny, charming, nice, easily distracted, and in the end not the guy for me. But he was my first. My first kiss, my first cuddle, my first sexual partner – my first everything. More importantly, he was the first man to teach me that sex was a way out of my body hatred, that I could escape my body by allowing myself to *feel* it, instead of always seeing and touching it. But even that wasn't the most important thing Josiah did for me; he was also the first guy ever to hold my hand and make me feel that swelling in my chest, that feeling that I'm worth showing off, even just to the strangers on a quiet shopping street. And that feeling was what cracked me wide open, what made me realise how badly I wanted a boyfriend, and how much I needed to share my life with someone.

If it weren't for Josiah, I would have continued feeling in my heart of hearts that nobody would ever want to be that someone for me. But even though *he* didn't want to be that person, entirely, Josiah did show me that it wasn't crazy to think that person might exist for me, somewhere out there in the great big world, and that my body wouldn't always be the first reason for someone not to want me romantically. It might take me a long time to find the right guy for me, but I felt calmer about it, somehow – just knowing that I was wrong to think my body was completely unlovable was comforting. And in the meantime, as I now knew, there was sex; some people would be willing to have it with me, and I could use it to escape my body issues for five minutes (or longer, if I got really lucky).

Before I met Josiah, I had no idea that my body could be good for anything – to me, it was an enemy, to be fought until I was too exhausted to fight any more, at which point I was forced to tolerate it. But now I understood that my body could also be a vehicle for something enjoyable, both physically and emotionally, and I was finally looking forward to exploring that enjoyment, in any way I could. And hey, maybe if I kept adding to the number and diversity of people judging my looks through their actions – choosing whether or not to help me escape my body through sex – I could balance the scales a bit, and maybe even begin to tip them against the lone judge who had been controlling my body image for as long as I could remember: me.

8

Tanzania, Africa, December 2004–January 2005

My legs are aching, and the soles of my feet burn from the heat of the dry Serengeti floor. I dodge another pile of buffalo poop and wipe my forehead with the tail of my shirt. Ahead, on my right, Andrew jumps over a fallen acacia branch, the dust rising in clouds where his feet land. With some effort, I catch up to him.

'Dude, it's fucking *hot*. Do you know how much farther it is?'

Andrew shakes his head. He doesn't look much better than I feel.

We've been walking for over two hours (a change from the usual long days in the jeeps), pausing now and then for water breaks – an hour ago we stopped at the school where the nearby Maasai kids learn to read and write, a building made of smooth, fist-sized stones piled on top of one another and bound with thin reeds. Now we're miles from any sort of man-made structure, surrounded by grass and dust and acacia trees. Up ahead, the guides glide over the dry earth, graceful and unconcerned; their tyre-sandalled feet hardly seem to notice the rocks and grass clods and roots that we stumble over so easily.

The necklace I bought yesterday – made by a local Maasai woman and beaded in bright yellows, greens, and reds, with horseshoe-shaped metal bars forming a yoke at the centre – is sticking to my damp collarbone, irritating my skin. All day the metal has been absorbing the sun's scorching heat. I pause to adjust it, and Andrew stops with me, crouching in the sparse shade of an acacia. He looks woozy.

'Hey, you OK?'

Andrew shakes his head slightly, but he says, 'I'm fine. Just hot.'

I don't believe him, but I nod anyway and start to move on.

'Well, hopefully we'll be there soon. And didn't Peter say there was water there we could swim in?'

'Yeah.' Andrew hauls himself upright. 'I keep thinking I see it but then it turns out to just be heat waves.'

The land is shimmering, as it has every day since we arrived. There are wildebeest everywhere; the world's edges are ridged with their awkward bodies, all humpbacks and horns. There are gazelle too, Tommies and Grants, mostly, and thousands of zebra, but this morning they're all keeping their distance. The only animals I can see are the ones that make up the bumpy horizon, wavy with heat.

Andrew is staring off into the distance too.

'Dude,' he says, 'I feel like I'm trippin' balls.'

'Seriously? You took shrooms, in *Africa*?'

'No, dumbass! Obviously I'm not stupid enough to bring drugs to fucking Africa, *fuck*. No, I just *feel* like I'm trippin'.'

'Um . . . are you OK? Do you want me to get Mom?'

Our parents are behind us, probably chatting with Peter, the owner of the safari company, or with one of the other guides. The rest of our thirteen-person party has split into smaller groups too, most of them clustered around a guide asking questions or stopping every few hundred feet to take photos or look for birds with their binoculars. I'm surprised to see Andrew flagging so badly – I thought my dad and I were the only ones suffering. Even after losing all his excess weight, my dad is still badly out of shape because he never has time or inclination to exercise, and although I try to work out regularly back at Washington University, I've been slacking this winter, preferring to curl up in my bed with a mug of tea rather than do biceps curls in the student gym. My mom and her sisters are exercise freaks, so this walk is nothing to them, and everyone else seems fine too. Except Andrew.

'No, I'll be OK. It's just weird.' As he says this last part, he starts wiggling his fingers in front of his face, and I start to worry.

'Don't be stupid. You probably have heatstroke or some shit, and if you let it get any worse *I'm* certainly not carrying your ass home.'

I march off toward my parents, who are currently arguing over who to assign to which jeep for tomorrow's game drive. Our guide, Peter, looks relieved to have a distraction from the conversation.

'Hey guys, um, Andrew's not feeling so great. Do you guys have any water or anything?' I drank all my water, and I know Andrew won't have brought any from camp. *Classic male thoughtlessness.*

'Is he OK?' My mom immediately heads in the direction I came from, her eyes creased with concern. I trot after her.

'Yeah, he's fine, he's just kinda . . . dizzy? I dunno, he said he was *trippin'.*'

I hoped she'd snort and roll her eyes, like I'm doing, but instead the lines at the corners of her mouth deepen, and she speeds up.

'Don't worry,' says Peter, striding confidently alongside us. My heart flutters at his proximity and I try to quiet my panting. I have a bit of a thing for him – a touch of 'khaki fever', my sister and I call it – and I don't want him hearing that I'm out of breath.

'He'll be fine,' Peter continues, 'he probably just didn't drink enough water this morning. We'll take a little break, and then we'll press on. We're almost to the spring anyway.'

'I *told* him he should have taken a bottle of water when we left camp.' I try to sound concerned instead of smug, and Peter smiles at me.

'Yes, well, we'll get him sorted out.'

Andrew is trudging up ahead, and when he sees us coming toward him he flashes me a glare and raises his palms.

'I'm *fine*, you guys, Annie just overreacted. I just have a headache, is all.'

Mom puts her hand on his forehead and Dad shoves a bottle of water at him. Andrew takes it and downs it in one go. I try not to feel envious – since the surgery, chugging liquid like that almost always makes me throw up.

'Peter, do we have any Tylenol or anything?' Mom is still looking worried, but she relaxes when Peter produces some small pills.

'Here,' he puts them in Andrew's hand, and passes him another bottle of water, 'take these and rest for a minute. We're nearly to the spring, and we can have some lunch and a bit of a swim when we get there.'

I try not to show my relief – I've been powering through this walk, across flat, arid land which started out cool in the early morning and heated up with a vengeance half an hour in. I've tried to hide my exhaustion, because I still feel like I can't show physical weakness or my physical flaws will become all the more glaring. Losing a hundred pounds doesn't mean I'm skinny enough to pant. Andrew can trip all he wants, but until I'm too dizzy to see straight I have to keep going, or the jig'll be up: they'll know I'm the fatty, the fall-behind, the one they have to slow down for and – worst of all – pity.

*

We hear the rush of water about twenty minutes after we've started up again, and Peter turns to me and grins. I'm glad for the camouflage the heat provides; my face is already so flushed that my pleasure at being singled out doesn't show.

The group has gathered closer together now, picking our way through the gurgling water that seems to bubble up from beneath us, less a uniform river than a long, wide stretch of moving wetlands. Green tufts of grass have burst up under our feet, and our hiking boots sink into the soft, wet ground if we're not careful. This new terrain slows us down, and more than once I wind up knee-deep in mud and sludge. Just as I'm really beginning to lose patience with the landscape, we arrive at our destination: the spring. It's not so much a clearly defined pool, but rather a wide, flat opening in the wetlands we've been trudging through. I slow down and catch my breath; the only sounds are the rush of the crystal-clear water all around me and the wet, sucking noise of my sodden left boot when I pick my foot up and set it back down again.

Peter turns around and addresses the group, waiting for the stragglers to pick their way over to him. 'This is a ground-spring; the water flows in from a deep mineral source underground. Some of you said you wanted to take a quick dip? Well, here we are!'

My dad is already whipping off his shoes and rolling up his pants, and I quickly follow suit. I pull off my boots and right sock, then peel off my soaked left sock and stick my feet in the water. It's cooler than the air, but not at all cold. Unexpectedly warm, really – and so soft, almost slippery without being oily.

I look down at my pants: zip-off, quick-dry hiking trousers. *Fuck it*, I think, *we'll be driving home anyway, and nobody around here cares about the gross image of my saggy ass and lumpy thighs with wet cloth plastered to them.* I zip off the lower half of the pants, set them on top of my boots, and step all the way into the spring. My dad grins at me.

'I like the way you think, kiddo!'

Soon, there are four of us in the water, up to our necks: me, Dad, Andrew, and our family friend, John. We're all wearing our shorts and button-down, long-sleeved safari shirts in different colours – blue, yellow, green, orange – like a bunch of Easter eggs bobbing in a river pool in the middle of the Serengeti. It's bizarre. It's amazing.

The water slips and slides around us, rushing gently over our tired legs and buoying our spirits. I feel the exhaustion and heat drain out of my body as the water flows over it; I turn to call the others in and see Catie, sitting on a tuft of grass with her *kikoy* hitched up around her thighs, her feet and calves in the water, her camera in her hand. She's shooting me. I should put my hand up to the lens, as usual.

But, weirdly, I don't. Instead, I smile, a big, wide, toothy, laughing smile. I feel the joy and ease of this wonderful land pour out of my face, and I imagine the photo: a tired, pink-faced twenty-year-old, having the time of her life. I even feel kind of . . . beautiful. For the first time since I can remember, I turn toward the camera, encouraging, posing, enjoying the attention. Catie grins at my rare enthusiasm and clicks away.

*

Africa made me feel something I'd never experienced before; looking out over the vast landscape, dotted with nothing more than acacia trees and four-legged herbivores, I was completely isolated, in a good way. I felt un-judged, and so I felt less of a need to judge myself. Every morning, I woke up in a tent, my breath clouding in the blissfully cold air, and dressed for the blazing heat that I knew was just an hour or so away. I wore unflattering, lightweight hiking pants; an

African cloth called a *kikoy* wrapped around my ass like a towel, topped with a yellow North Face fleece in the mornings; my favourite jersey skirt and flip-flops. We spent most of each day inside the jeep, so even though my parents had harassed me for weeks before the trip to buy all kinds of 'activewear' at the local sports store, I ended up in whatever was comfortable. And I was comfortable – the jeep was roomy and the people I shared it with were old friends and family members, so there was nothing to remind me that I should be thinner, firmer, or at least better accessorised.

I didn't care about my appearance at all. I never put on makeup, and barely did my hair. Most days I just pulled it into a ponytail and tucked the wisps behind my ears. The rare evenings we spent at lodges or hotels, I felt like a wild thing that had been brought into someone's home to be domesticated: on edge, bristling, desperate to get back out to the plains, my tent, and the campfire circle. On New Year's Eve, we stayed at a luxurious lodge, and had a big, extravagant dinner, and all most of us could talk about was when we'd get back out to camp, to our bug-covered dining tent and our camp chef's salty peanut soup and goat's cheese salads. We'd been in Africa for a little over a week, and we were all falling in love, fast and hard. Other people annoyed us; if we ran into another jeep on a game reserve, we rolled our eyes at each other and commented on how embarrassing the 'tourists' were. We weren't tourists, in our minds – we were becoming a part of the land.

Of course, this was ridiculous. We were on an extravagant safari, just like the rest of them. The guides we thought of as our friends were being paid to chat with us about the gestation period of baboons and how to guess the age of a baby elephant (if it can still walk under its mother without touching her belly, it's under four weeks). But we ignored our rational knowledge that we were just like any other tourists; we, and especially I, clung to the *feeling* that Africa gave us, that we were all just humans, like any others, and nothing else mattered.

I had backpacked through the Joshua Tree desert, wound my way through the souks of Morocco, been all over western Europe and sailed the coast of Croatia; I'd been travelling all my life. But this was an entirely different experience; it was the first time since I was a little kid that I just let my body be a body and nothing more. It was there to transport me from place to place, and food was a necessary (if exceedingly delicious) fuel. My ass was for sitting on, my boobs irrelevant, besides their high risk of sunburn. My belly, covered with loose button-down shirts or peeking out of tank tops or even bulging a bit out of my skirt if I got up too fast to see an animal, was just another part of the vehicle for my heart and mind. Life wasn't about rolls and jiggle and pasty, unshaven legs; it was about the migration, the land scattered with herds of wildebeest, zebra, and gazelle. Life was the hunt for a cheetah on the chase; the search for the elusive leopard; a cup of tea and a card game around the campfire before dinner. It was the huffing of a lion outside my tent in the middle of the night.

Life was all around me, and for once, it had nothing to do with *me*.

To me, those two weeks in Tanzania meant a vacation from society – any kind of society – and therefore a break from myself. I had a tendency to project my own concerns about my looks onto everyone else: the lady in the supermarket who looked at me funny must have been wondering if my breasts were really that uneven; the waiter who watched me as I passed by the window of his restaurant must be thinking about how weird and square my butt looked when I walked; the little kid who couldn't stop staring at me on the bus must have been hoping he'd never *ever* get that fat. But in Africa, those worries barely crossed my mind. I was with twelve family members and friends, plus four guides, mostly older men and all more interested in nature and anthropology than my hip width. The only judgements on my appearance would have to come from the animals, and besides the lions thinking I looked like an easy kill and a week's worth of meals for the whole pride, I couldn't imagine they gave two shits about me. And that invisibility was the most freeing feeling in the world.

This isn't to say that every single day in Africa was an escape from my insecurities. Of course I had moments where I felt fat or out of place, but they were few and far between, and the anxiety they created was shockingly fleeting. A self-conscious moment about my hip hanging over the edge of a camp chair was almost instantly replaced by laughter at my aunt Nancy losing very ungracefully at a card game; a 'fat morning' of dressing was instantly forgotten in the steam pouring off my mug of tea; a roll of belly flab was hard to focus on when, just outside the jeep, lion cubs were pouncing on each other. It wasn't that I never felt bad about myself, but rather that it was hard to stay mad at my body when it had so little to do with the rest of the world, and the rest of the world was so startlingly fascinating.

I was beginning to understand that my body was more than just an object to be gawped at by some people and scorned by others; it was a fabulously able vehicle for exploring the world. Trekking through the Serengeti that day was hard, but it was also beautiful and peaceful and gave us a whole different view of Africa than we usually got from the jeeps. Until that day, I don't think I really appreciated how capable my body was, and had always been – having a fully functioning form allowed me to travel in ways that let me really connect with new lands and people. I hadn't understood just how lucky that made me until I tromped through the desert with one wet boot squelching beneath my aching feet. And I'm not sure I ever could have seen my body as so useful if it hadn't been for the removal of the societal pressure to view my body as more important for how it looked than how it performed. Of course I still worried about my body and my appearance – I refused to wear pants unless the day's activities required them, preferring to spend jeep days in my soft, jersey skirt that covered my belly overhang; I still tried to swallow my panting when anyone was near me on a hike; I ate fewer digestive biscuits than I wanted to, tempering my intake to match those around me – but for once I had to acknowledge that the pressure was all in my head. I couldn't blame the outside world, because the outside world didn't give a toss about my body so long as it could perform properly, and that meant my own self-inflicted anxiety carried less weight.

The day we left Tanzania, flying in a teeny-tiny plane back to Kenya for our journey home to the US, we all took lots of pictures with the staff and said goodbye to each guide. As the wheels left the ground, tears rolled down my face. I cried for the experience I was leaving, the new friends I felt I'd never see again, and for the stunning landscape with which I'd fallen so deeply in love. But mostly, I cried because I knew I was going back to myself. In escaping 'normal society' for two weeks, I'd somehow escaped my projections of my own scathing criticism. But it couldn't last for ever, and I was terrified of the world I was going back to, a world of self-loathing and insecurity. I'd had a taste of what some lucky people have always known – unselfconsciousness – and I was greedy for more.

Unfortunately, I was right about Life After Africa, as I came to think of it. Back at school after the winter holiday, I fell into a deep depression; I spent afternoons 'napping' in my single room, hiding away from my roommates. I would come home from class and shut the door and crawl into bed, sometimes falling asleep right away and sometimes just lying there, bundled in my warm jersey sheets, under my heavy, flannel-covered duvet, staring at the map on my wall. Wishing myself back to Africa.

All the fear and hatred of my body that had affected me before the trip came flooding back with a vengeance, and I withdrew from everything that had previously distracted me from myself: friends, school, extracurricular activities. All I wanted to do was mope and sleep. And nobody could help. My best friend, Emily, who lived in the other single room in our suite, was going through her own drama with her long-term boyfriend, and she spent much of her time in her room with the door closed as well. My other close friends, who lived in the double room next to me, did their best, inviting me to hang out with them and listen to music, and, when I refused, knocking on our shared wall every now and then to remind me they were there. But I wouldn't budge. I was mired in sadness and self-pity, and I couldn't bring myself to try to get out.

Until, one frozen evening in early February, I decided it was bullshit. With much effort, I hauled myself out of bed and Googled 'home cures for depression'. I ate a banana, the only item in my room that was on the list of 'mood foods' I found, and as I mashed the soft flesh with my tongue I realised I hadn't really enjoyed eating anything for weeks, not even the sweets and cookies I'd been slowly (and normally, excitedly) reintroducing into my diet in small amounts and even allowing myself to use as a comfort sometimes, although never to a pathological level. Since the surgery, I rarely got really *hungry*, but I did feel a desire to eat, whether because my stomach felt kind of empty or because I was lightheaded and cranky, or just because food looked or smelled or sounded delicious. Even though just the thought of things like fried foods and rich desserts made me feel ill, I still had cravings for milder sweets or salty snacks or particular meats and vegetables. I had finally been allowed to enjoy food without so much baggage, and I was loving it. I tucked into salads and steak and broccoli and Oreos with equal gusto, depending on the day's desires, and even as I had to watch my consumption of sweets and fatty foods, it finally felt like I was being careful for the right reason: because I cared about my body and how it felt. It wasn't so much about other people's perceptions or expectations any more. I was finally free to love food without fearing that the world would see me as an obese glutton.

So that day when I realised that there was no food I could think of that I actively wanted to eat, an alarm bell went off: *If I don't enjoy food any more, even chocolate, then I may as well be dead.* When I realised that literally *everything* I enjoyed – reading, hanging out with friends, writing, and even eating – was unappealing to me, I decided that I was more than just 'sad' or missing Africa: this feeling was like all the bad days I'd had in my life, days where I felt sad and listless and hopeless for no apparent reason, only this time there were weeks of them, all in a row. I was a mess, and something had to be done. The banana was the first step – it seemed crazy to believe that something as easy as eating a banana could make me feel better about my location, my body, and my whole life, but I was willing to try anything. The next suggestion was to take some physical steps; I needed to get outside and go for a walk.

I wasn't completely immobilised by my sadness. I was walking to and from classes every day, which was a good half-hour round trip, but I wasn't really moving much. I was trudging. Shuffling. Getting from point A to point B because I knew that skipping class simply wasn't an option.

But I hadn't just gotten out and moved around, and paid attention to the world around me, in weeks. Part of my excuse for that was the weather: St Louis in the winter is pretty damn cold, and often snowy and icy. It was easy to go inside, get in bed, get warm, and stay there. It also wasn't unusual. The cold was a convenient cover for my real reason for staying in.

But now I called myself on my own bullshit. I got up from my desk, took off my pajama pants and put back on the jeans I'd discarded on the floor earlier. I threw on a sweater, pulled on my sneakers, and ran a brush through my bedhead. Coat, gloves, hat, ready. Journal and pen. I barrelled out of my dorm before I could lose my nerve or anyone could ask where I was going.

I was going to the suburbs. Wash U is in suburban St Louis, surrounded by surreally idyllic residential areas, where pretty two-storey stone and brick houses perch on immaculate lawns and shine a warm light through the front windows onto the streets below. Streets where little kids play, where young couples jog together, where teenagers walk their neighbours' dogs. Streets that were empty at eight o'clock on that weekday night, but for one wandering college student. Everyone else was sitting down to family dinners, or more likely cleaning up from family dinners and sitting down to family TV time.

I strode down dark, snowy sidewalks, trying to force my heart to work harder, to pump the blood through my body and a little life back into my mind. I peeked in windows, made myself notice the sting of cold on my cheeks and nose, the sound of my footsteps crunching on the snow. For the first time since our plane took off in Africa, I focused on the world, the smell of ice and burning wood, the taste of banana still lingering on the backs of my teeth. I walked to the seminary and found a bench, where I sat in the cold and pulled out my journal; I took off my right glove, uncapped my pen, and wrote some very bad poetry. I think I used the term 'souls of their shoes' to describe the young men, studying to become priests, who passed me and smiled kindly. And I laughed at my bad poetry. And then I walked home, a little lighter.

Until that day, I'd never believed that something as simple as walking could lift a person out of depression (and I still don't believe it's that simple, or that it would necessarily work for anything worse than mild depression and nagging sadness, like mine). I think the exercise was beneficial, and it certainly reminded me to appreciate the usefulness of my body outside of how it looked, but what really pulled me out of my depressed state was the world outside myself. That's what I had missed so much about Africa – in Tanzania you can't escape the vastness of the earth, or how little it cares about your jiggly ass, even if you try – and that's what I had failed to find again in St Louis. But I hadn't been trying hard enough.

Because St Louis was the world outside me too, as was San Francisco or any other city or country – any place besides a small room with a closed door. And *that* was what the trip to Africa taught me in the end: not that I could escape my self-criticism and body anxieties (or at least temper them) in the middle of the Serengeti, although it was certainly easier there, but that the key to escaping my cruel inner self was looking out, at new places, new experiences, and new people. That revelation was to be the beginning of a whole new kind of travel for me; from then on, rather than taking myself on vacation, I would travel to take vacations from myself.

I'd been disappointed to find that having surgery and losing a hundred pounds didn't completely 'fix' my body – I was still bigger than I wanted to be, and now I had an abundance of excess skin to contend with. Even worse, though, the weight loss didn't even come close to vanquishing the bitch in my head: that nagging critic who constantly harped at me about my body, my social skills, my incurable singleness. Still, I couldn't just concede the fight. The surgery set off a series of battles, some of which I won (I could now fit into clothes in normal stores, barely), some I lost (I was still the largest person in most rooms, and I still sat gingerly in new pieces of furniture because some part of me was still afraid I weighed too much and would break them), and some I would have to continue to fight. And the more weapons I had, the more ways I could find of either beating my inner bitch or at least ignoring her for a time, the better off I was in the long game. That was where travel became more than just a fun pastime – it became a useful tool in the battle against my worst critic, a tool I discovered only after I went to Africa and lost myself there.

From then on, I would go to new places to flee my own self-judgement and to learn new, positive things about my body that I could add to my arsenal and use in the fight against my self-hatred. And when I couldn't travel outside the place where I was living, I'd just have to travel within it.

9

Milan, Italy, June 2005

'See, now *that's* a woman.'

Becca is eyeing the painting appreciatively. *Jesus, she's eye-fucking a painting*, I think, *how hard-up* is *she?* But I blush as she turns and slides her gaze up and down my body, the same smug, approving look on her face. I keep my eyes focused on the canvas in front of us: it's a run-of-the-mill Italian oil painting of Adam and Eve in the Garden of Eden. They're completely nude, and completely innocent; in Eve's left hand she's holding the apple from the Tree of Knowledge, but neither of them has taken a bite yet. They look content, and in love, and none the wiser. I envy them their ignorance.

'Hm, yeah, she's hot,' I muse, keeping up the pretence that it's Eve's body we're analysing. 'I mean, she's not exactly perfect by today's standards, is she? But it's interesting how much more *realistic* their desires were back then.'

'Yup, because *curves are awesome.*' Becca grins, her dark brown hair falling into her olive-green eyes as she looks up at me. I ignore her hinting tone and try not to think about how pretty her eyes are.

'No, but I don't even mean that. I feel like she's not so much *curvy* as she is . . . muscular? Strong. Look at her stomach; she's got like an eight-pack! Yeah, sure, it's got a layer of fat over it, but what really gets me is how in these paintings it matters more how strong the women are than how gorgeous. Or they're the same thing, to these painters. Of course they all have perfectly round, symmetrical boobs and beautiful faces, but instead of being delicate and waifish, *fragile*, they're robust and almost as muscular as the men!'

Becca is nodding, but she's also blatantly staring at my very imperfect, asymmetrical breasts, which are mounding up a bit out of my cheap tank top. I tug on the neckline and adjust the shawl around my shoulders and keep talking.

'Did you ever see pictures of the Garden of Eden scene in the Sistine Chapel? Eve is almost as muscly as Adam! It's crazy. I wonder if that was really considered attractive or if Michelangelo just painted them both kind of similar, as just *humans* rather than male and female. Does that make sense?'

'Yeah, I think so . . .'

I'm not sure she understands what I mean, and I'm not sure I care anyway. I stare up at Eve's body, her small, round breasts with their tiny pink nipples, her muscular haunches with nary a dimple in sight, her soft lower stomach, pooching out a bit beneath her belly button, the crease where her hip rounds up to meet her waist. I put my hand on my own hip, covered in the soft, stretchy skirt I've been living in this summer; I feel my body curve in the same way as Eve's, but then I let my hand slide down my side to my outer thigh, more saddlebags than strength, mushier than they are muscular, and I sigh and turn away. *Maybe I should show pictures of Eve to that plastic surgeon I'm meeting next month ... I wonder if he can make me look as firm as she does.*

Becca is moving on down the line of paintings and frescoes along the church's west wall, pausing here and there to check out more of the nude female form and then breezing past. At the end of the room she stops and turns around, looking for me. I pretend I haven't seen her and drift over to the shrine for St Anthony, tucked into the wall behind an iron grate; I recognise him from his plain brown robes and the chubby, blond child he cradles against his chest – the baby version of Christ. Fishing in my shoulder bag for my wallet, I see Becca wander up, feel her hand on the small of my back. I stiffen a bit as she touches the soft shelf of flesh above my ass, one of the body parts I absolutely despise, and shift so her hand is higher up, nearer my waist.

Becca frowns at my discomfort, but she just sighs and says, 'Hey, you almost ready? I could really use a gelato, and I think we've lost the others.'

I scan the floor of the cathedral; it's packed with tourists, and I don't see our friends anywhere. I shrug my shoulders, then go back to searching in my bag. 'Eh, they're probably in the gift shop. Or maybe they got bored and went outside.'

Becca notices my rummaging and leans in closer to me to look in my bag.

'Whatcha doin'?'

'I want to light a candle for –' I pause. *Do you really want to know? Are we seriously going to have a conversation about my uncertain faith or my need for rituals to calm my anxiety? Can I actually talk to you about my cousin who was taken from us when he was far too young or my grandmother who died just as I was beginning to feel there was someone in my family who really understood me?'* – It's just this thing I like to do at the churches I visit. Makes me feel . . . peaceful.'

Becca's eyebrows go up, but she backs off.

'Look, why don't you go find them and I'll meet you guys outside in ten minutes? I know you're all kinda bored of churches, but I just want some time to sort of soak up the atmosphere, you know?' I smile and shrug my shoulders as if it's no big deal. *No reason to confide in her too much – she's already got far too much power over me.*

Becca looks sceptical, but she shrugs too.

'Yeah, whatever, just don't take too long. I'll miss you!' She shoots me a wicked grin and her hand slides down, just for a second, over my ass. I do my best not to react, although a small shudder runs through me at the flashback to last night, outside the bar, when that young Tunisian guy put his palm in the exact same place. But his was inside the under-pants. I reach around and pull Becca's hand up, giving her an admonishing look that's gentler than my internal reaction. *We're in a fucking church!*

'Don't worry, you'll see me soon enough. Go get some gelato and do some people-watching in the piazza and I'll catch up with you as soon as I'm done here. Won't be too long.'

'You better not be – we need to make sure we have plenty

of time to get ready for the clubs tonight.' She bumps her hip against mine and I wince as a wave of jiggle crosses my body. 'You are gonna *love* the gay bars!'

I laugh. 'Yeah? You aren't afraid of some predatory lesbian *turning* me?' Becca goes a little pink, and I enjoy having the upper hand in our game, even though I know it won't last long. She leans in close to my ear, her hand sliding over my hip now.

'I'm not worried,' she whispers, 'I know the only person who could ever turn you is me.'

With that, she finally takes her hand off me and backs up a bit. I roll my eyes at her, smirking at the suggestion that I would ever go for someone like her, then we both turn away from each other. She heads toward the exit to find the rest of the group and I light my candle, then move off to find a slice of quiet in this so-called sanctuary.

As I walk farther into the cool, dark recesses of the church, I sneak a look over my shoulder at Becca. She's striding toward the front of the church with the same overconfident walk she uses out on the street and, no doubt, on the softball pitch. From the back, she looks like a short, stocky teenage boy with a thick brown ponytail, but from the front she's too pretty to be mistaken for a man, and underneath her cargo shorts and tie-dye T-shirt are a small, firm waist, curvy hips, and soft, heavy breasts.

I know, because I've fondled them.

*

A few weeks after finishing my second year at university, little more than a month after my last date with Josiah, I found myself on a flight to Italy. I'd started taking Italian lessons the previous fall to supplement my English major and my Spanish minor, and I loved the language, so I'd leapt at the opportunity to study abroad for six weeks in the summer. But by the time the departure date rolled around, the friend who had intended to go with me had discovered she couldn't make it and I was terrified to go alone. I nearly backed out. If it hadn't been for the draw of my favourite (so far) European country, I might have opted to stay behind. Instead, I convinced myself that I was no longer the fat outcast I had always forced myself to be – isolating myself and avoiding parties for fear of shunning and humiliation that never came – and even allowed myself to believe I might make friends. So I left my parents on the outside of the security gates at San Francisco airport, took a deep breath, and got on the plane.

I was shaking when we landed in Rome. After twelve hours of folding myself into the smallest person I could be and suffering through the dry, cold air, crying babies, bloat-inducing airplane food, and other people's smells, I was ready to be on the ground, but I was in knots with anxiety about meeting my group. I wandered through the airport, through customs and immigration, hauling my big pink wheelie suitcase and keeping my red eyes peeled for the little cafe where we'd been told to wait for our teachers. Finally, I spotted it. There was one other person my age there: a good-looking black guy in jeans and a T-shirt, sitting in a plastic chair with a big suitcase pulled up next to him and iPod headphones in his ears. He looked up when I approached, and smiled, taking the headphones out and reaching his hand out.

'Hey, you here for the Wash U programme?'

I took his hand and nodded. We introduced ourselves. I sat down in a chair next to him and tried not to think about the width of my hips spilling over the narrow frame.

And that was it. The social stuff was so much easier than I'd expected. It turned out that very few of the other students who'd signed up for the trip had come with friends in tow, and those who had were happy to add to their little groups. I made friends easily, friends who didn't seem concerned with the size of my jeans or the sagginess of my upper arms – the kind of friends I'd been lucky to have all my life, really. Within hours we were chatting like old chums, telling each other about our families and whispering secrets about our sex lives (a conversation in which I could finally participate honestly). I loved them all, harder and faster than I'd ever expected.

But the one I loved most was Becca. We clicked immediately, and we wasted no time becoming close. We bunked together, staying up late to talk about the relationships (or 'whatever', as I called my thing with Josiah) we'd left behind; we sat together in class, writing notes on each other's papers and getting shushed by our long-suffering teachers; we studied together at little cafes on the outskirts of town, drinking cappuccino after cappuccino and practising our Italian with the baristas. And we travelled together on weekends, when we'd leave the hostel in Arezzo to visit Rome, Milan, Pisa, Florence, and anywhere else within range.

Becca made me laugh. She was goofy and silly, but she could also be serious and intellectual. We spent hours talking about her experiences as a young lesbian – the difficulty of coming out to her parents, the emotionally draining relationships she'd gotten herself embroiled in, and the political stands she made on a regular basis to ensure that she never allowed herself to be treated as a second-class citizen. We also spent a lot of time talking about me. Once I'd told her about my history with weight and the surgery – after a particularly sticky pasta dinner at the hostel had me throwing up in the bathroom all night – the floodgates opened up. I felt more comfortable talking to Becca about my body-image issues than I had with anyone I'd met in years; I told her the details of the GB and my reasons for doing it, and we talked about the ways the results had elated and disappointed me. I admitted my fear that I'd never lose any more weight, my concern that I would never be happy with any weight – a concern I was just beginning to understand – and my hope that an upcoming appointment with a plastic surgeon would at least help me understand what could and couldn't be changed about my body. She listened to all of it without judgement, and when anyone else in the group unintentionally made me feel uncomfortable about my body – when the girls would ask why I never wanted to go shopping, for example, and I would awkwardly dance around the admission that even after the GB there was still no way I would fit in any Italian clothes – she stuck up for me, causing diversions and changing subjects like an old pro. She cracked jokes, and made sympathetic noises, and generally made me feel understood, and I loved her for that. And then, as we got closer, she began to make me feel something completely new: alluring.

By the time I met Becca, I knew I wasn't so hideous that *nobody* would have sex with me – Josiah had disproven that fear – but I still felt unattractive. I guess I saw myself as not completely *un*fuckable, but someone for whom nobody would make much of an effort, based solely on looks. Sure, Josiah had made the effort to flirt with me and ask me out, but he hadn't gone much farther without my prodding him, and anyway I figured any energy expended on his part was in pursuit of my face (which was always pretty enough, even when I was fat) and a passive acceptance of my body. Even in the bedroom, Josiah had seemed sort of generally aroused, rather than being turned on by me, specifically. And I was OK with that I didn't expect anything more. But Becca had a preoccupation with my *body*, of all things; even before I told her what I'd gone through with my weight, she had already made it clear that she found my form not just passable, not just acceptable enough to ignore while she focused on my face, but actively *attractive*.

Still, I was straight, even if I refused to label myself as such, and so for weeks I simply took her comments about my shape as empty compliments from a friend, and later, once I'd told her about the surgery, I figured she'd upped her compliment game to help boost my self-esteem. I allowed her opinion to carry a bit more authority, though, if only because she was into girls and therefore would know better than I would what was sexy in a woman. Sure, she would tease me about my 'undefined' sexuality, challenging me to prove that I wasn't straight and telling me all sorts of intimate reasons why she loved women instead of men, but we never crossed the line from flirtation to action.

All this time, though, I was feeling pretty lonely; I didn't exactly miss Josiah, but I did miss having *someone*. I'd been given a taste of what it felt like to have someone's hands on me, to have someone kiss me and want more, and I wanted more. I *needed* more, needed someone to want me, to provide some sort of argument against my own opinion that I was completely unwantable. I felt cheated by Josiah; I'd finally gotten rid of the VIRGIN stamp on my forehead, and all I got out of it was a tiny bit of sex and a lot of angst. I'd been to Italy before, on my trip after high school with Andrea and Courtney, so I knew how forward the Italians could be, and I was ready to return their advances for once.

But instead I found Becca. She was a far cry from the man I thought I wanted, but she was also someone I could trust, and anyway I was open to trying new things. I saw no reason to limit myself to the term 'straight' – I come from an open-minded family, and I went to an all-girls middle school where most of us experimented at least a little bit, so I wasn't concerned about setting boundaries before I'd experienced enough to know what I wanted. But, until that year, I hadn't experienced much at all. I'd kissed girls, but only straight girls, usually at sleepovers as a dare, and until Josiah I'd had zero experience with boys. Once I'd pushed past that first barrier, I figured, I might as well barrel my way through them all. 2005 was to be my year of taste-tests.

There was something intriguing about her, and it wasn't just the fact that she was a girl. On the contrary, Becca seemed more like a teenage boy: she was cocky and loud, walked with a little bit of a strut, and was obviously thrilled by the chase. I was the only person in the group even remotely interested in playing her game – all the other girls were straight and definitely knew it – so teasing me became her favourite pastime. And I can't say I didn't enjoy it too, most of the time. I loved getting hit on by Italian guys in front of her. She got extremely jealous, even going so far as to push one of them off me at a bar (which I appreciated, because he was taking too many liberties and I didn't have the guts to stop him). One night, in Venice, a cute waiter actually left in the middle of his shift to buy a rose from a hawker out on the piazza and bring it to me at the table, in front of the entire group. I turned as pink as the petals and agreed to try to make it to a nearby bar to meet him at 11 p.m. I never went; I was terrified to go alone, and I knew Becca would ruin it if I brought her. But I didn't mind too much – the possessive way Becca stuck by my side the next day was worth any missed make-out opportunities.

I missed a lot of opportunities that trip. For all my psyching myself up and convincing myself that it was a necessary benchmark on the road to adulthood, I was nowhere near ready to have a random hook-up with a stranger. Especially a sexually aggressive stranger, which a lot of the Italian men I'd met were. Even the best-looking ones were so intense and in-my-face that I backed off immediately, and Becca turned out to be a worthy ally in that. Not only did she keep the guys off me in clubs and bars, she replaced some of the attention I would have gotten from them, which made it easier to say no. I liked Becca – she was blunt and straightforward and crude, like me – and I liked the way she looked at me, like I was a prime cut of meat. Becca was the first person I'd ever known who eyed me with a sort of hunger. Even when he was getting down with it, Josiah was pretty passively appreciative of my body, but Becca actually *dug it*. And I dug that. I had never felt so desired in my life, and I loved it. It provided a great retort to the bitch in my head who kept telling me I was still fat and therefore worthless: *If I'm so gross, why is she so desperate to keep me for herself, even when she's not getting anything out of it?*

So when Becca stopped being just a friend and started to flirt with me in earnest, I decided she should get something out of it. I was missing the affection Josiah had taught me was available (if only in limited supply), and I was curious. We still didn't cross the line into sexual contact, but our 'friendly' hugs got longer and, er, *friendlier*, and our conversations nudged at boundaries we thought we'd set.

A couple of weeks before the end of our programme, our professors took us to the beachside party-town of Rimini for the weekend. We hung out on the beach all day, just relaxing and chatting. Becca and I even rented a jet ski – of course she drove, while I clung to her waist like the wussy girl I am and tried not to scream (I failed). But at night we let loose. All day on the beach, hot young girls and guys walked up to groups like us and tried to entice us to come to their nightclubs later on. They offered transportation and free drink tickets, and we gladly accepted. We went to massive, multi-level clubs and danced and drank and laughed, and then we would return to the hotel and crash, or keep drinking on the beach. Which was exactly the setup Becca and I needed to cross the line.

I don't even remember much about that night, besides a lot of tequila and a lot of making out. I do remember one of the guys in our group seeing us and running back to tell everyone what we were doing. I also remember a weird, three-headed creature making out with itself in the waves off-shore: the three gay boys had decided not to leave anyone out of the fun. It was just another wild, drunken night, and we all wrote it off as such, but things changed between Becca and me that night. From then on, every time we were alone, we would steal kisses or gropes. I felt my first boob (besides my own, obviously), and got the appreciative touch I'd been craving as well. I noted how different kissing her was from kissing Josiah; where he'd used a lot of tongue, Becca used almost none. I actually found myself wishing she would use it more.

It was weird, and embarrassing, and exciting. A couple of my friends took me aside to warn me that she was just head-fucking me (was I that obviously vulnerable?) and everyone in the group got a kick out of watching our little drama unfold, but I was so caught up in the game that I mostly didn't care. The thrill of having someone chase me, even in such a sideways, secretive manner, was too much fun. Becca's strategy was clever, and it worked: she would act like she knew better than to hook up with me (I was straight, and she was sure of it even if I wasn't), but then she would come after me anyway, as if she just *couldn't resist my body*. It was intoxicating.

Just like in Africa, it was hard to hate my body for long when I was surrounded by so many distractions – and when I did feel that self-consciousness creeping up inside my throat, I had a support system. Having Becca there to fancy me meant that seeing other people hook up or get hit on didn't send me into the usual 'Why not me?' downward spiral. For the second time in my life, I was able to enjoy travelling without worrying about what other people thought of my body; this time there were plenty of people around to judge me, but I was protected by the knowledge that someone I liked thought I was gorgeous. I thought of Becca as the perfect friend-with-benefits; I was quickly realising that I preferred men, which meant that I couldn't be hurt by her not wanting a relationship, but physically she was a great stand-in for the moment. It seemed ideal to me.

Once it came time to leave Italy, though, I realised how emotionally invested I'd become in my new friends, especially Becca. I cried like a little kid on the flight home – I felt like I was leaving behind the best parts of myself, the fun, almost carefree person I'd allowed myself to be while I was in Italy. I missed Becca – only as a friend, but I cared more about her than I'd planned. It was Life After Africa all over again: I was losing a sense of place, leaving a location that made me feel like I could truly relax, and I was also leaving a whole new group of wonderful friends, including the first person who had ever made me feel like my body was an asset rather than a liability.

I knew it was silly to get so upset; we were all going to be back at the same university in a couple of months. And the rest of the summer would be fun, spent with old friends and family – I also had the meeting with a plastic surgeon to look forward to, and maybe I could even get something done about my saggy body. But the sinking feeling in my ribcage turned out to be right; when I got back to school that fall, I rarely saw my new friends on campus, and we all grew apart quickly once we reunited with our 'real' friends. Even Becca and I barely saw each other. We hung out a few times, but I found her changed in the presence of her softball buddies and prospective girlfriends. I didn't matter as much to her, and so she came to matter less to me.

Nonetheless, the change she had effected in my self-image stuck around; every time I saw her on campus, or passed her in the cafeteria, I noticed my hips swaying a bit further from side to side as I walked, my movements a bit more exaggerated. I felt myself get slinkier, and I *used* my body instead of trying to hide it. I couldn't say whether she noticed the change, or even noticed me, but *I* noticed. Becca and I had had something special, a close friendship, but I had enough friends that I eventually got over that loss. What remained was the important stuff: the memories, the new experiences, and, most importantly, the knowledge that, for a few strange people out there in the world, my body was something to be *actively desired* rather than simply overlooked.

If Africa was my escape from societal pressures and my

own self-consciousness, Italy was my safe haven from my thoughts about what might have been with Josiah and whether my body was the reason nothing more came to pass – between my flirtations with Becca and the attentions of the lascivious Italian men, it was also a break from feeling like the least attractive girl in the room. In travelling, I had again learned something new about my body: not only was it useful for tasks like hiking through the desert or climbing cobbled streets in hilly towns, but it also had its advantages in the relationship game, which I was finally learning to play. I was beginning to understand that as much as *I* still found it disgusting and frustrating and embarrassing, my body was genuinely attractive to some people, and the simple presence of that knowledge gave me hope that maybe even I could actually like my figure, some day in the far-off future. If only I could pile enough positive external views of my body on the opposing scale, maybe one day I could balance out all the hateful, negative feelings I'd been cultivating about myself.

It was worth a try, anyway.

10

St Louis, August 2005

My arms are sweating. Not my underarms, because the nerve damage there means no sweat or hair for a while, but my upper arms, where my biceps lie hidden beneath stretchmarked skin and long red scars. It's at least ninety-five degrees outside, and the air is so humid it feels like it's resting on my face, but I'm wearing a sweater with sleeves past my elbows. I need it to cover the pressure garment I've been wearing since July, when my new doctor sliced a twelve-by-four-inch piece of skin and fat from each of my inner arms.

I run my right hand over the inside of my left arm to see if the sweat is bad enough to send me inside to take refuge in the air conditioning; I finger the edge of the sleeve, checking to make sure the bumpy scar that runs from armpit to elbow isn't peeking out. At the movement, Emily looks up from her book and smiles, then turns her head away from me again, her gaze travelling over the huge oval of grass we call the Swamp. She bops her head and swings her legs to Jason Mraz on her iPod.

I adjust myself on the blanket that Emily has spread out

for us, settling my weight on my left hip and arm and bending my legs to the right. The movement pinches my skin at the top of my waist, where the elastic from my control-panel granny panties digs into my flesh. It's causing rolls on my hips, too, where the leg openings are, and I say a silent prayer of thanks for the stiff, thick cotton of my dress. *One thing I will say for plastic surgery*, I think to myself as I smooth the bright pink material from my hip down to the hem, where it meets a layer of white cotton peeking out by my knees, *it helped me fit into the adorable dress I've had hanging in my closet for a year!* I slide my hand back up the skirt, pausing at the multicoloured polka-dot ribbon that encircles my waist, and up over the bust to run my fingertips over the same ribbon, trimming the strapless neckline. My fingers linger, savouring the difference in texture between starchy cotton and silky synthetic, then they move up my chest to my collarbone. Their favourite place to dance, playing over the hard, hollow bone and firm, deep dip, revelling in the way the depth changes as I breathe.

'Hey, Emily, hey, Anne!'

I'm startled. My hands fly away from my body as I look up and see John, Josiah's best friend, and somehow always a presence in six degrees to anybody – the kid seems to sorta-kinda-know pretty much everybody I meet, even though he's not a student any more and it should be weird that he hangs around campus so much. I force a smile as Emily takes out her earphones and sits up.

'John! Hi!' She smiles brightly, always genuine. I shift my

position a little to ensure that no granny-panty rolls are poking through the cotton. 'Want to sit?'

She scooches over, and so do I, carefully. I try to arrange myself on the blanket to take up as little space as possible, hyper-aware of the obvious difference between Emily's teeny bottom and my sprawling hips. I glance over at John as he settles beside me. *God forbid he sees anything unflattering and reports back to Josiah.* But then I notice that he's smiling at me in a way he never has before, and an entirely new thought crosses my mind. *Oh my God, maybe I look* good. *Maybe he'll report back that I've gotten more attractive and Josiah made a huge mistake!*

My smile turns genuine, and suddenly I'm pleased to see him.

'So, John, what're you doing on campus?' I ask. 'Helping somebody move in?'

Classes haven't even started yet; Emily and I and our roommates are just getting settled into our third-year dorm, where we'll be staying for a semester before we all scatter around the world for study-abroad programmes in the spring.

'Nope,' he grins, 'just visiting friends.'

I try not to roll my eyes. *You're always visiting friends. Maybe you should get some friends your own age.* I force a false smile and nod. 'That's cool. Emily and I were just taking a break from unpacking. I'd almost forgotten how great the people-watching on the Swamp is! Last year we lived in the Sophomore Suites, so we never really crossed the Swamp.'

John nods, and I blush, as we both avoid acknowledging

how he knows where I lived last year; not only did Josiah and I have sex in that dorm, but John dated a girl who lived in the next building over, and I would sometimes see them sitting on her patio. *Usually when Josiah hadn't called me back, and I had to restrain myself from going over and yelling at John to set his friend straight.*

I wave my hand in front of my face in a feeble attempt to move the air, and wince a bit as the tight scar in my armpit pulls a bit. 'Jesus, it's hot as fuck out here.'

'Yeah.' Emily stands up. 'I might need a drink. Anybody want anything?' She pulls her ID card from her shorts pocket and waves it around.

I request a Powerade with a grateful look and John shakes his head but thanks her anyway, and she bounds off toward the student centre, her long, slender legs carrying her fast over the grassy Swamp. I try not to think about my own legs, stumpy and blubbery under my dress, and to reassure myself that it's not all bad I allow my hand to wander over my newly flat tummy. I can't feel the hands stroking my belly – the skin there is still numb – but my palms relish the smooth, taut surface.

I turn back to John and rack my brain for something to say. 'So, how was your summer?' *How was Josiah's summer? Did he find someone new? Was it the girl he hooked up with when we were still seeing each other?*

'Eh, it was OK. Hot. Man, I miss college, though, when summer meant three months off instead of just hotter days and the same old work schedule.'

'Ick, yeah. I'm definitely not looking forward to having to

deal with the real world, with a real job and only *two weeks* of vacation a year.'

John makes a *gee, thanks* face and I try to look apologetic and refocus my blather to something less depressing for him. 'God, and I don't even know what I want to do as a career – not that being an English major helps. Whenever people ask me what I want to use my degree for, I tell them it's qualified me for nothing and everything, so I have no fucking clue. The more I think about it, the more I lean toward teaching, if only because they get so much time off . . .' *Are you still seeing that girl, the weird one who pretends we've never met? Do I look hotter than I did last time you saw me? Can you tell I've 'had work done'?*

We sit in silence for a while, the sun punishing my pale skin and causing my nose to sweat. I look around for anyone else I might know, or something interesting to comment on. The cicadas fill the quiet with their rasping noise. Finally, just as I'm about to make some inane judgemental remark about the outfit on a girl passing by, John speaks.

'So what are you doing with all your studenty free time? You do anything fun or exciting this summer?'

I hesitate for a split second before deciding not to tell him about the surgeries. TMI – Too Much Information. Instead, I focus on the early part of the summer.

'Well, I went on an exchange programme to Italy, which was awesome.'

John raises his eyebrows as if he's interested, but I don't really want to talk about Italy right now – I miss it too much. So instead I ramble on.

'Other than that, though, not much. Although two of my roommates did come out to visit me in San Francisco, which was great.' *Except for the fact that I couldn't drive because I was on Vicodin, and I couldn't swim because I was in bandages, and I could hardly walk anywhere without my stomach killing me.* 'I mostly just chilled with high-school friends and spent time with family and stuff. It's always good to be home, but I was definitely ready to come back.'

'Yeah, it's funny how that happens. By my junior year I was dreading going home for Christmas break every year.'

'Well, it's really weird for me, because I was *so* homesick freshman year, and even last year, and I still haven't shaken it but now it's like I'm homesick for Wash U when I'm home, and I miss home when I'm here ... I'm starting to feel like the older I get, the more people and places I gather to miss when I'm away from them. Does that make sense?'

'Yeah, I think so.' John smiles thoughtfully, and I realise that maybe he's not as weird as I thought. Maybe he just misses college, and being on campus makes him feel like he hasn't completely severed himself from that part of his life. *But why am I even telling him all this? It's not like I got this personal, emotionally at least, with Josiah ...*

'Yeah.' I lean back on my elbows and look out over the Swamp. There are three different Frisbee games going on, and a couple of girls in bikinis have laid out towels and are now sunning themselves on the cement 'beach' across the Swamp – I allow myself a brief moment of fantasy to imagine my body as less-than-hideous in a bikini when it heals, but then I'm swallowed by the now-familiar fear that I'll never be normal no matter what I do, so I shake my head to try to rid myself of my anxiety and go back to looking outward. The pathways are starting to get crowded now as more kids head to the cafeteria for lunch, and people are running into each other and catching up, doing the 'how was your summer' all over the place. It's peaceful, and despite the throbbing in my arms and abdomen I feel more comfortable here now than I ever have.

'Helloooooo!'

I turn my head and see Emily's gangly legs striding up the slope of the lawn. A plastic bag full of bottles swings from the crook of her arm, and the cup of frozen yogurt in her hand is melting over the sides and onto her fingers. I sit up to take something from her, but she just plops down on the blanket next to me and starts licking the melted fro-yo off her hands.

'Oh, no!' She's dripped it on her shorts. She shoves the cup at me and starts trying to clean herself up, and as the sticky, cold goo dribbles down in between my fingers I start to laugh. Pain shoots across the lowest part of my abdomen, and I can feel the sleeves of my sweater creeping up my arms as I shift the yogurt cup from hand to hand, but for just a minute I don't care about any of that. I just laugh, and watch the bikini girls, and smile at John, and finally let myself believe that maybe this time all my insecurities have been sliced off and slipped into the medical waste bin along with all that excess skin.

*

Six weeks after I got back from Italy, a month after my initial meeting with a plastic surgeon, I went under the knife again to remove some of the excess skin my weight loss had left behind. I wanted to have it all done in one fell swoop, but the doctor said it was too risky to have the skin pulling in all those directions at once, so I settled for arms and stomach first, and legs two years later, the summer after graduation. I had also wanted the full body lift – a belt incision around the entire midsection, which pulls up the ass as well as tightening the tummy – but he didn't think I needed it. I stood there at that initial meeting, naked except for the smallest undies I owned and an open paper vest, and kept my mouth shut. He was the expert, and I was trying to learn to control my expectations. He pushed and pulled, poked and prodded, rearranging my skin as he hemmed and hawed. Then he looked up at me, like a sculptor who had successfully assessed the block of marble before him, and smiled.

'OK, Anne,' he said, 'I think we're going to get a great result here. See, I think I can get about four inches of skin from your arms' – he pinched a large chunk of my right bingo wing – 'and probably a good eight to ten inches from your abdomen here.'

I looked down at the hanging, wrinkled skin drooping over the elastic in my underwear, and thought about how it would feel to have all that flesh be gone. *Ten inches!* I tried to imagine looking down at a normal twenty-year-old's stomach. I couldn't, but I was excited. I was also secretly thrilled that he'd suggested a bit of liposuction to 'smooth out' the areas he would be rearranging. I knew it wasn't just skin dangling off my body like old cheese off a lasagne – it was fat too, but I was afraid to admit it. I still couldn't quite believe that the gastric bypass hadn't made me lose all my fat. Worse than that, I'd put on about ten pounds in the past two years, which made me start panicking about gaining it all back again. I knew it was possible, and the doctors had warned us to be aware of our weight and not expect it to stay down without effort from us, so I was trying to do my part. It was down to me now – my parents weren't around to encourage me to go to the gym or to stock the fridge with healthy food. I was on my own, and I intended to prove to them that the surgery was the leg-up I needed to fix my problems on my own, which meant *not* gaining the weight back through laziness and dorm food. I'd been working out, and trying to pay close attention to my diet, but it was so hard to see any subtle changes in my body; in addition to wanting the excess gone for my own self-esteem, I was also hopeful that if I could get rid of it I'd be able to see the results of my efforts better, and thus stay motivated to keep going.

I had a lot riding on this operation.

Standing before the doctor, my bare feet freezing on the tile floor, my naked breasts grazing against the paper vest, I learned new things about my body. I learned it wasn't my fault the skin was so loose, that I was right to suspect that all the exercise in the world wouldn't fix it, and surgery was the only option; I learned that my butt wasn't as drastically saggy as I thought, and maybe a whole lot of squats would fix that; most interestingly, I learned that my body's unevenness *was* noticeable to other people. Even more so than I'd realised.

'Now, everyone is asymmetrical, Anne,' he grinned up at me, holding the vest out to the sides so I was fully exposed, 'everyone has one foot bigger than the other, one breast larger than the other, and your left hip is a bit larger than the right as well, so we'll need to lipo a bit more of that and even you out.'

Wait, but you said the boobs were uneven! I KNEW it. Everyone's been lying to me. I didn't even know my left hip was bigger, but all I cared about was that he'd fix it for me. I wanted him to fix my breasts too, but I was afraid to become a different kind of monster altogether: one of those women who can't recognise when they've had more plastic surgery than common sense would dictate. So I stayed silent and just nodded.

After the topless show and the subsequent and equally humiliating 'before pictures' were over, I put my clothes back on and went out into the accounts office to talk money. My mom sat next to me, trying not to show anxiety over her youngest child going into the hospital for the second time in five years, not to mention how much this would all cost. I wished I could avoid this part and just have the surgery without knowing how much my parents were spending. I wished I could turn to my mom and tell her it was fine, that I didn't need this to be happy.

But I did need it. I was sick of looking in the mirror and seeing the same hideous beast I'd seen before the surgery, only this time smaller but aged about forty years, and deformed. I couldn't take it any more, and I think my parents understood that, even my mother, who tried and failed to hide her disapproval of my choice to have elective surgery *again*. I'd grown tired of defending myself: I felt like I was always telling her that exercise wouldn't affect the tautness of my skin; repeating over and over the evidence I'd read that skin doesn't shrink back; shoving photos from *People* magazine's 'Half Their Size' articles between her reading glasses and her *New York Times* crossword, pointing and insisting. 'Look, see? She lost the weight slowly, through diet and exercise, and she's *still* got that saggy thing going on with her arms and thighs! And see? Here? She says she's considering plastic surgery to get rid of it.' Eventually, she gave in, probably more because she was tired of hearing about it than because she really understood just how tortured I still was by my own body. But I wasn't picky; I didn't need complete understanding, just agreement, a chequebook, and someone to pick me up from the hospital.

So I went under anaesthesia again, and my parents paid for it *again*. I felt even guiltier than I had before – I couldn't tell myself this surgery was a necessity. I was doing it for vanity alone. Not that my motivation for having the gastric bypass was anything other than the intense desire to fit in and be normal, but that wasn't obvious; I could always keep my mouth shut and let people assume I did it for health reasons.

This time, though, it was obvious why I was having surgery, and this time I went in on my own. Not that my dad didn't talk about doing it with me. When I told him what I wanted to have done, his response was the usual: 'Sign me up!' But he was already well into middle age, and for all his normal vanity and love of quick fixes he wasn't interested enough to make this one happen for himself. A little sagginess in the belly and throat wasn't such a big deal for an older man; it was expected, and his brain and bank balance would always be more closely tied to his self-esteem than his body ever would. Anyway, he wasn't willing to take the time off work required to recover from major surgery again.

And it did take time. It took longer than I expected, and much longer than recovering from the GB. I had to spend the night in the hospital so my pain could be controlled by morphine, injected into an IV in my foot because my arms were too delicate to mess with – not that it helped my pain much when the night nurse depressed the needle so fast the liquid burned through my veins all the way up my leg. I didn't call for morphine again until I thought she might have finished her shift, and boy did I suffer for it. I lay in a sort of half-sleep that whole night, drifting in and out of an anaesthetic haze, waking up when the nurses chatted outside my door in the echoing hall or someone came to check my vital signs or empty my drains.

Yup, drains. I had three of them, in my abdomen. The space my doctor had to clear so he could pull my skin down was so large that they needed to put these plastic tubes inside to make sure everything drained properly. The tubes snaked through my torso, from the top of my ribcage down to the incision at my bikini line, ending in three little plastic squeeze-balls, with openings kind of like the blow-up bit of a pool toy. After I left the hospital I had to empty them myself; they would fill up with blood and a yellow liquid I could only assume was pus, and the smell was putrid – sweet and sour and sticky. It wasn't how I'd pictured spending my summer, but I told myself it was worth it.

And it was, eventually. After a week, the drains were removed – and what a *weird* feeling that was, having a long rubber tube pulled through my stomach just under the skin, travelling all the way from just below my left breast to my right hipbone – and I was allowed to take a shower. That was my favourite day of the entire month. The worst thing about recovering from the plastic surgery wasn't the pain; it was the smell. By the third showerless day, I was so sick of smelling like *wound* and being unable to do anything about it that I had a total nervous breakdown: my parents had a meeting with their architects, and I had quarantined myself upstairs while they convened downstairs at the kitchen table, but just as I was beginning to believe that I was safe, one of the architects was struck with an urge to use the bathroom, which, of course, was upstairs. I nearly pulled my stitches hobbling from the couch to my parents' bedroom, her heavy footsteps on the stairs urging me forward as my chest closed in panic. I sequestered myself in there, sobbing and terrified, for an hour before my mother impatiently convinced me that their guests had left. In general, I got little sympathy from my family, who spent most of their energy staying as far away as they could from my self-inflicted disgustingness. I could hardly blame them (although I still did).

Once I could shower and the drains were removed, I started to feel a little more human. I was still a cripple, though; for weeks I couldn't really go anywhere. I had to walk hunched over, nearly bent in half by the tension in my abdomen. I was irrationally terrified that if I stood up straight, the two-foot scar that ran across my hips would rip open and my guts would come spilling out. But I was too self-conscious to walk around like an ancient crone in public – my mom eventually had to ban me from seeing movies with my friends because I would come home in excruciating pain, having walked through the theatre with my back held as straight as I could get it, pain be damned. I was put on house arrest until I could move a bit more normally.

Two weeks after my surgery, two of my roommates and close friends from university flew out to San Francisco to visit me. I had assumed I would be recovered enough to show them the city and hang out with them, but I was wrong: I couldn't even drive because of the pain medication I was on, much less walk around for hours on end. I did my best to think of low-impact activities, and my mom was kind enough to drive us around, but I doubt they felt they'd gotten their money's worth from the plane ticket, and I was a nervous wreck. When they left, I breathed a sigh of relief and sat curled up on the couch for two days straight.

And the pain wasn't the only thing I had to worry about; because of the liposuction, my body retained a ton of water and I was extremely bloated. You'd think this would have upset me, but I was actually kind of thrilled – for a brief and beautiful period of time my skin was taut and firm. To ensure that the bloat didn't get too bad, though, and that the remaining fat (and there was plenty) on my body redistributed correctly, I had to wear compression garments –

made of thick, elasticated material that was *required* to be worn too tight – for months. My mom took me to a medical supply store and bought me some fancy sleeve things so I wouldn't have to constantly rewrap the bulky Ace bandages around my arms, and we also got a foot-wide elastic band with Velcro at the ends, to wrap around my abdomen on days when I just couldn't handle the granny panties, which were actually kind of cute. They were from Hanes, and had a lace overlay on top of the super-tight stomach panel. They looked very vintage: low leg opening, high waist. I didn't always hate them, but sometimes I was driven to the edge of madness by all the rolls they caused at my hips and waist. The elastic band was better under clingier fabrics.

I wore the compression garments for at least twenty-two hours a day, for three or four months. Every time I went back for a checkup, I would beg my doctor to let me take them off, but he held firm. When I was finally given the OK to go without them for a few hours every day (I had to be weaned), I actually kind of missed them. I'd forgotten what it was like to feel my arms jiggle, and I didn't like it. But I was thrilled with the results. Sure, my hips were still squishy, my thighs and ass still sagged, and my body overall was still bigger than I wanted it to be, but for a little while my focus shifted from hating everything below my collarbone to loving my stomach and arms, and trying to ignore the rest as best I could. It was easy enough in those first few months to focus just on my new body parts; they hurt, which demanded attention, but they were also visually distracting.

I had three long, angry red scars on my body: one on each

arm, running up under the armpit and down to the elbow, and one running across my lower abdomen like a sadistic Joker's grin. It took months to recover fully, and even years later I still feel twinges of pain if my scar is pinched by a seat-belt or someone squeezes me too hard around the hips or the waistband of my jeans gets too tight. But it was worth it; for the first time in my young adult life I felt a little bit *normal*. I would catch glimpses of myself in a window in the months after the surgery and I would stop to admire how flat my stomach was from the side. I joined my school gym and worked my arms relentlessly, until I could see a line of defin-ition curving along my biceps, just under the scar. I waved at people on campus, even when I was wearing a sleeveless shirt, without keeping my elbow pinned awkwardly to my side.

Those first few months after the tummy tuck and arm lift, I was the most confident I'd ever been. And, foolishly, I even thought it might last, that the plastic surgeries really had fixed *everything*. But I would eventually realise that they had only fixed my excess skin, and even that only on my arms and stomach. There were still plenty of body parts for me to hate, and I would soon discover that I could always find something to be unhappy about.

11

Rome, Italy, April 2006

I should have had more dinner. Or less wine at dinner. The room is dark and a little wobbly, and I feel like I might fall off my high bar stool if not for Guy's hand on my knee. I grab my €7 Corona and take what I hope will be a stabilising sip. The lime revives me a little and I look around to get my bearings, blinking hard.

The bar, all stained wood and corners, is the third (or maybe the second?) on the pub crawl organised by the Roman hostel where I'm staying for two nights with my friend Kelsey from my study-abroad programme in England. We got to the first place right before open-bar ended, just in time to down two double screwdrivers each, which mixed a little too well with our dinner of picked-at mixed salad and a litre of house red. So far my semester abroad has been less about studying English literature and more about making friends with American sorority girls, travelling all over Europe whenever we get the chance, and drinking far more than I ever did back at Wash U, even after I turned twenty-one last December – I'm enjoying pretending to be more social than I actually am, so when Kelsey drinks, I drink, and the screwdrivers were no exception. The boys, three barely legal Brits from our hostel room, were already well into a colour-coded drinking game by the time we caught up with them, downing some green concoction that made my stomach turn. Before I could understand the rules, though, we were whisked to the next spot, and then this one, and the next thing I noticed was the warm, sprawling hand on my leg.

I look at him, *really* look at him for the first time since we met this morning. He looks young, sure, but with that gingery stubble he definitely doesn't look eighteen. He's kind of handsome, in a non-pretty-boy, clever-but-masculine way. Silvery-blond hair parted kind of preppily, wire-rimmed glasses, pretty nice teeth for a Brit. Tall. Sweet. He's smiling at me, that huge, guileless grin, and saying something about how much he likes the Red Hot Chili Peppers – 'Dani California' is playing over the speakers, and I nod my head vigorously, then quickly regret it as the room sloshes in the corners of my eyes. I swallow my momentary nausea and try to recover with a story.

'You know, when my sister was younger and she worked in Oakland, there was this hot guy that worked at the cafe next to her store, and he looked just like Anthony Kiedis, you know, the lead singer? With the long hair? Not Flea. He's the drummer. Or the bassist? Anyway, she took me over there to get lunch and I said something really loudly like "Oh yeah, he *is* cute!" and it embarrassed the shit out of her.' I'm so tickled at the memory that I start to giggle. Guy smiles even wider, and his hand moves a little farther up my thigh. He leans in, close to my ear.

'I really like this dress on you.'

I blush. *Of course you do. Between the neckline and my cheap H&M push-up bra, I'm surprised I haven't smacked you in the face with a nipple yet.*

'Um, thanks. I don't really think it looks very good on me. My friend is like half my size and she has the same one, and of course it looks awesome on *her.*'

He frowns as if he doesn't understand and pulls himself up straight.

'But you've got a *great* figure!'

I giggle again, this time at his accent: *fig-aah.* I shake my head and scoff under my breath, but I leave it at that. *Remember, the plan tonight is to pretend to be normal. So just shut up and smile.* We sit in silence for a minute, and then I realise we're alone.

'Hey, where are your friends? And my friend?' I scan the room for blonde curls and spot Kelsey, in the corner with Tom, the tallest of the three boys, the slender one with the reedy charm. She's hitting on him, blatantly. I turn to Guy to share a laugh at our friends and he kisses me, hard, and with tongue. I'm shocked, but I kiss him back. *What the hell? Why not have a random hook-up? I guess he wasn't just being nice about my fig-aah . . .*

A bit of kissing and a drink or two later, the hot Italian guy who works at the hostel, and who's chaperoning all of us tonight, stands up and announces that the bar is closing. We're welcome to stay out, he says, but if we need to be led back to the hostel he'll be leaving in five minutes. I look at Guy.

'So? Back to the hostel?'

He leans in, running his hand up my thigh and over my hip (I try not to flinch as he grazes the dimpled flesh), and whispers something about preferring to stay here with me. I think for a second, and then put my mouth close to his ear.

'I have condoms at the hostel . . .'

I do. I packed the motley collection that the Wash U health centre gave out months ago. I mostly brought them in case any friends of mine needed them – babies and STDs aren't in my friendship contract – but I'm not averse to the idea of using them myself. I just didn't think anybody would be this interested in wearing one for me.

But Guy is definitely interested. Once he's recovered from the shock of my shamelessness (I'm still reeling a bit myself), he tucks the evidence of his interest into his waistband and pulls me off the stool and into another sloppy kiss. *He could definitely use some practice . . .*

We walk out of the bar with Kelsey and Tom. By this time they're holding hands, and Kelsey and I give each other *go for it* looks, then take our respective hook-ups aside and make each promise that his friend is 'a good guy'. So promised, we hug and part ways.

*

'And that's kind of where I blacked out. I mean, I remember, like, stumbling over cobblestones, and kissing on the corner of the street, but after that, nothing. Until I sort of woke up . . . in a park . . . on my back . . .'

On the other end of the line, back in the States, Courtney gasps. I'm chewing my thumbnail so hard I'm afraid I might rip it off. I glance up at the window of my hostel room, where Guy is still sleeping off last night's debauchery. The sun gets in my eyes and I choke back vomit.

'Wait, you had *sex* with him in a public park?!' Courtney sounds somewhere between appalled and impressed.

'Well, no . . . not *sex*, exactly . . . according to Bill Clinton.'

'Oh my God, Anne, you gave him a BLOW JOB in a public park?!'

I wince at her un-minced words.

'Shh! No! It was more, like . . . receiving . . .'

'WHAT? Oh my God. That is *amazing*.' Courtney is laughing so hard I have to hold my cell phone away from my ear a bit. When I woke up and texted Courtney about my crazy night, I never thought she'd go so far as to call me, in ternational, but I guess that's just how crazy this all is. *And how good a friend she is*, I think, feeling all warm and fuzzy for a second before I feel pukey again. She's still laughing, and I try to bring the focus back to the story.

'Shut up! I don't even know how I got there, I just know I had twigs in my underwear when I showered this morning.' I touch the toes of my flip-flop to the edge of the sidewalk, pointing like a ballet dancer and testing my balance.

Courtney can barely breathe, she's laughing so hard at me. I try to be mad at her insensitivity to my embarrassment, but I'm smiling too. It's just too ridiculous.

'I know. I *know*. I feel like such a ho.' The thought of my-self even having the opportunity to be a ho tickles me.

'So?' Courtney has recovered enough breath to ask for details. 'How was it?'

'Um...' I shift my weight, and my nether regions burn. 'It was ... terrible. Courtney, seriously, it was so *painful*. I don't know *what* he was doing but I'm, like, *crippled*. Maybe he used his teeth? I don't know, but I was faking it so hard just to get him to stop.'

Courtney sucks air through her teeth in an expression of vaginal sympathy.

'Why? Why why *why* would he use his teeth?!'

'I don't know! It was bad. But he was super drunk, so maybe he just wasn't paying attention.' I pause for a second. 'Oh, guess what *really* bothered me, though?'

'What?'

'OK, how fucked up is this: when I realised he was, you know, *down there*, it didn't upset me what he was doing, not nearly as much as the realisation that he had to *pull down my tights* to get access!'

The other end of the line is silent; I feel like I can hear Courtney trying to figure out what I mean. *Damn.* I was hoping she would get it right away – after all, she's the one friend I can usually talk to about issues like tights-roll and back-boob. But she's not following this one. I try again.

'You know? When you take tights off? And the fat kind of... spills out?'

'Oh my God, Anne, you're insane. Obviously he likes your body, or he wouldn't have been all up in your grill.'

'I know, but I just hate the way it all comes pouring out, like I've opened an overstuffed sausage casing...'

'Ew, thanks.' Courtney's laughing again. 'Wait, though, he *crippled* you! Can we focus on the important stuff here? What happened after he crippled you?'

'Well, that was like two in the morning . . . so after that, I guess we got up to try to head back, and then we got *so* lost. I mean, I don't think I've ever gotten that lost, anywhere. It was crazy. We crossed the river like three times, and I know we ended up at the Vatican a couple times because we were sort of grinding on each other against the wall and I kept talking about how we were going to hell . . .'

'Classy. I bet the pope was watching you guys from his bedroom window.'

'Ew! Creepy. Anyway, we wandered around until like five a.m., just walking and kissing and talking. At one point, it was so cheesy, I said the moon looked really beautiful, and he was all "*You're* really beautiful –"'

Courtney makes a gagging noise, and I laugh.

'I know, right? I was like, "Not as beautiful as yooo," in a dorky voice, but I don't think he got that I was making fun of him. It was so weird, he kept telling me I was *hot*. I was so uncomfortable. I just kept waiting for him to come out of his drunken haze and realise that I'm too fat to be hot.'

'Anne. Shut up. Clearly, he's attracted to you, because he was all over you –'

'I know! I kept telling him he'd already sealed the deal and he didn't have to lie, but –'

'Woman! You are ridiculous. Anyway, what happened after that?'

'Well, at five or whenever the sun was coming up, I looked

in the canvas bag I'd been carrying around all night? And I realised I had a map in it.'

'NO.' I can imagine how wide Courtney's round hazel eyes are right now.

'YES. I know. God, I must have been so plastered. I mean, I've never blacked out before in my life. So we realised we had a map, and we'd been going in circles, and we figured out the way home but by then my feet were killing me, like, my skin was peeling off they were so rubbed, so I hailed us a taxi, which Guy totally didn't want me to do because he was out of money and he felt so bad letting me pay.'

'Aww, what a sweet little teenager you hooked up with!'

'Shut up. But yeah, he does seem sweet . . . Although, this morning he looked so miserable, and I slinked out of his bed all shameful, 'cause I was terrified he'd woken up, seen me, and been full of regret for hooking up with a fatty. I mean, he was completely turned away from me, toward the wall, and his face was all scrunched up . . .'

'Anne. Stop. So did you guys have sex in the end?'

'Ha! No. Poor guy – poor *Guy*, hehe! By the time we got back to the hostel it was six a.m., and we'd been wandering around all night, and I just wanted to go to bed. So I asked if I could just sleep in his bed with him, and we cuddled up and passed the fuck out.'

'Awww Anne! That's so cute!'

'Yeah, if you ignore the part where I was trashed and had my ass out in a public park.' I cringe and slap my forehead. *Oh God, ow.*

'Hey, it happens to the best of us!'

'Yeah, right.' As far as I know, Courtney has never had sex, oral or otherwise, in public, but it's kind of her to pretend.

'So what do you think is going to happen? Do you think you guys will keep in touch?'

'I don't know. I mean, they're staying until tomorrow, and so are we, so I might give him another shot tonight . . . but I don't know if I'll be up for anything in the down-theres, if you know what I mean. All I can say is I am *so* glad I brought Neosporin with me, otherwise I don't know how I would walk around Rome today.'

'Eeesh, poor you! Was he at least a good kisser?'

'Umm . . . He was . . . passionate. He did kind of slobber all over my face a bit . . . but he's just a kid! And anyway, who am I to say? I mean, nobody's ever complained, but then again there have only been two of them before now!'

'I'm sure you're a good kisser. I feel like girls are naturally better at it than guys.'

I laugh.

'Hm, maybe. Anyway I don't know where this might go, but I'm kind of liking the idea of it being a random hook-up. How perfect would it be if my first random hook-up was with a guy named Guy?'

'Pretty perfect, I'm not gonna lie.'

I smile. *Perfect. Now if only I could get rid of this hangover*
. . .

We chat a bit more, then say our goodbyes and hang up, and for a moment I just stand there on the sidewalk, breathing in the cool, shady air. I take one more look up at the green wooden shutters of our hostel room, willing Kelsey to come down so I don't have to go back in there. And for the first time ever, she seems to read my mind. She comes flouncing out of the building and grabs me, making my head and the entire street spin nauseatingly.

'Oh my God, Anne, what *happened* last night? We definitely need to talk.'

*

The day I met Guy, one of the first things he did was offer me chocolate. He stood there on the linoleum floor of our shared hostel room, holding out a melting bar of Lindt milk chocolate, the red wrapper ripped haphazardly across the middle as if the idea of wrapping it back up and saving some for later was madness. He looked at me and said, 'Oh, go on.' Just like that. As if it were nothing.

I demurred; the idea of taking something so obviously sinful from a boy I didn't know was beyond the realm of possibility. I was so stressed out as a result of my morning journey into Rome that I didn't even do the usual mental dance of trying to figure out his intentions – *Is he trying to trick me? Does he assume I like chocolate because I'm fat? Is he just being polite?* – I just shook my head, smiled, and went back to trying to shove my overstuffed backpack into one of the lockable drawers under our shared bunkbed. He shrugged, licked a glob of chocolate off his finger, grabbed another forty-ounce bottle of beer from his own drawer, and left the room.

It's sort of amazing that I didn't jump his bones right then. I mean, usually all it would take was a little flirting and the barest hint of possible attraction to make me think of any guy as a potential boyfriend, and here he was *offering me chocolate* and I wasn't even thinking (yet) about thanking him with a little making out? The only sensible reason for my lack of interest in him – besides my own frantic travel stress – was the fact that he was three years younger than I was, but even that hadn't been a barrier for a few of my past crushes.

By 2 a.m., though, I had changed my mind, both about his age and about hooking up with him. I could tell that Guy was different. There was something so serious about him; he certainly acted much older than any eighteen-year-old I'd ever known. Hell, my own brother was twenty-three at the time and he spent his days playing video games with friends and eating microwavable chocolate cake. And here was this boy, this *kid* whom I'd only just met and to whom I'd drunkenly offered myself like a cheap buffet, talking about how excited he was to go to university and study medicine, telling me stories of his early life in places like South Africa and southern France. It was kind of hot, but his intensity also freaked me out a little. In comparison to his heavy feelings about his parents' divorce or his stories about being a young teen in Sydney, my rather straight-and-narrow life path – childhood in suburban LA; teenage years in San Francisco; studying English at a good but not Ivy League university; doing a semester abroad in a country that's basically the US but with more drinking and less Mexican food – seemed dull, and if I could have such a boring background and still be as messed up as I was, it didn't bode well for this kid's sanity. I felt like he couldn't possibly be normal and be so interesting, and so *interested*. There was no way someone like me, with a dull background and beyond-imperfect looks, could have genuinely attracted a cute, smart, sweet kid like Guy – there had to be something wrong with him.

As a result I was a bit distant from him on my second night in Rome. The group of us from the hostel room – Kelsey and me, Guy, Tom, their horrible little friend Sam who hated Americans on principle rather than experience, and another girl who'd just arrived that day – went out for pizza at a little trattoria, where I sat between the girls and ordered too much, as I often did when presented with too many tasty options. I let my eyes and mouth win out over my wee stomach, and as a result I couldn't finish my pizza *or* the caprese salad I'd insisted on having as a side. That was when I learned the first great thing about younger guys: they eat a *lot*. The boys polished off my leftovers and I was spared the awkward explanation to the waiter about why I hadn't eaten more than a few slices of pizza and a chunk of fresh mozzarella.

After dinner, we all went for drinks, although I limited myself quite strictly. I wasn't one for getting very drunk in the best of circumstances, and although I had a relatively high tolerance (despite the doctors telling us the surgery would mean one glass of wine had the effect of four, my liver was apparently huge so that didn't apply), once I did get a little drunk the liquor would sneak up on me very fast. I'd learned my lesson the night before, so I had one mojito, which I didn't even drink because I'd forgotten how much

I hated rum. I didn't mind sticking to Coke, though; I was there to socialise, not get trashed.

But the socialising was a little weird. The whole evening, Guy kept reaching for me, grabbing at me. It was not what I expected from a hook-up, especially one that I'd written off as a drunken mistake on his part, and it was kind of possessive. I kept dodging him; I'd let his hand rest on my waist for a minute, then squirm out and go dance with the other girls while he watched me from the table (he refused to dance). It wasn't like he was being creepy, but seriously, who in his right mind would act protective of the girl he'd just hooked up with, especially when that girl was *so* not a catch he needed to worry about other men poaching? I didn't get it. So I tried to avoid facing it: I flirted with older Italian men and pretended to ignore his glowering; I waved him toward younger, slimmer girls, encouraging him to go have fun; I rolled my eyes with Kelsey when she asked why he was acting like my boyfriend.

It was strange. *He* was strange. I didn't know how to react to him – all I'd wanted was a little booty, and I assumed he wanted the same. But all of a sudden he seemed interested in more, and it weirded me out. More than that, I was kind of mad at him for ruining my first random hook-up. It was so perfect – a random guy, *named Guy*, a sordid one-night stand in Rome, an embarrassing but funny story to tell at parties – it was everything I'd been hoping for from my travels. I was finally starting to feel like a normal girl, who made normal if sometimes ill-advised choices instead of being forced by her body to play it safe. Even if I still felt disgusted by my body, still felt too big and too jiggly and too unattractive, my plan for this trip was to pretend I *didn't* feel that way, and let the boys decide whether they wanted me or not. Until I met Guy, I'd not had much luck on the one-night-stand front, so when I hooked up with him I was thrilled. But then he had to go and act like it meant something.

Which is probably why, when we parted ways two days after we'd met, I stood in front of him in the hostel lobby and shrugged my shoulders. I offered little more than a clipped 'Bye', operating under the usual assumption: *He couldn't possibly want more from me than he's already gotten, and even if he does, that's way too much effort for a fling.* We stood there like that for ages, the awkwardness thickening around us like custard, until Kelsey, bless her loudmouthed soul, broke in.

'Why don't you guys just *exchange email addresses*?' she asked, as if suggesting that we put one foot in front of the other to walk somewhere.

I shrugged again, and wrote my email address on Guy's smooth, muscular forearm with a ballpoint pen. *Best to leave it up to him.* I wasn't expecting anything – maybe a Facebook friend request.

Kelsey and I spent the morning wandering around Rome, and then we went to the train station together and got on separate trains. She headed for Spain to meet up with a couple of other friends from our programme, and I went north to Florence to stay with a guy friend of mine who was studying architecture there. On my second day with him, I went to his school to check my email and found a missive from Guy, talking about how much he missed my touch and how special he felt I was. I spent the next thirty-six hours obsessively thinking and nattering about the possibilities this presented: *Boyfriend? Prank? Fling? Good story for my blog?* My poor friend probably sprained an eyeball from rolling them so hard.

I wasn't finished with my European adventure yet, and after my experience in Rome I was no longer so certain that I didn't have any hook-up options out there in the world, so I was cagey in my response to Guy. I couldn't just ignore his email – he was sweet, if a little strange, and anyway that would just be rude. So I wrote back, saying I'd had a great time with him too and that I was glad he had emailed me. I told him funny stories about my visit to Florence, and wished him luck in his final exams at school. Then I signed off and went back to my travels.

After I left Florence and my friend behind, I was on my own. My plans hadn't fit with anyone else's schedule, but I was determined to see some new countries so I went it alone. I visited Vienna first – Andrea had been there on a music trip and she'd told me it was one of her favourite cities. I stayed in a hostel, where I forced myself out of my comfort zone and introduced myself to strangers; I met a couple of nice Canadian girls with whom I had dinner the first night, but then they moved on to Germany and I spent the rest of my time solo. And Vienna was a little *too* welcoming.

I'd arrived in the city on a high from the attention I'd gotten in Rome, and rarin' to flirt. But the men were way too up for it. Everywhere I went, I was hit on, and I was even followed a couple of times. One of those times, I ended up eating lunch at 11 a.m., just so I could duck into a restaurant and get away from the tall, dark-haired, Fabio-looking dude who'd passed me on the street and doubled back to follow me. I sat behind a pillar in the cafe and watched him enter the piazza outside, look around for me for a while, then leave. My heart was thudding so hard I thought I might throw up. After a few months of feeling like a normal girl, I was suddenly back to being the easy target, the fat victim – I felt like I didn't have any right to fight back, to confront these guys about their behaviour, because I was afraid they would just laugh in my face and humiliate me. I didn't feel normal any more; I felt singled out, and not in a good way.

When I got back to the hostel that day, I emailed Guy about what had happened. I didn't know why – I told myself that I needed a male perspective, or I just wanted to get in touch with someone in roughly the same time zone, someone who could reply before I went to bed. And he did reply, appalled and upset and concerned for my safety. I laughed a little at the intensity of his email, but I also felt a bit better. His email made me feel safe, like I had just as much right as anyone else to be upset and scared – he made me feel normal again. For the first time in my life, I found myself wishing for a man by my side for safety and security, and for some reason Guy was the person I wished for. I told myself it was just because he was the last person I'd hooked up with.

But I didn't stop emailing him, or wishing he were there. In Lisbon, at the castle fort on the top of the city, I sat and looked out at the bridge that so resembled my beloved Golden Gate, and I wrote in my journal about how much I thought Guy would like it there. And then later I emailed him about it.

We were becoming penpals, which was a nice change for me – my family is pretty crap at communicating, so it was rare for me to have anything but junk mail in my inbox. It was a disappointment to make the effort to go to an internet cafe in a foreign country, only to find that most days the only people who'd bothered to get in touch were DailyCandy and the Wash U Student Union. So when Guy and I started writing to each other, it was nice to open up my email and see a new message from a real human being. And I liked him; he was funny, and sweet, and goofy. He said nice things about me, especially about my looks, and even though he wasn't with me I could feel the effect his compliments had on my confidence as I travelled. I spent every day noting little stories or funny scenes so I could recount them to him later, and in return he told me about his weird dreams and suggested new music for me to download. It was fun, but that was all it was.

After all, he was just a random guy, just somebody I hooked up with so I could prove to myself that I *was* capable of a one-night stand, just like any normal non-religious girl. He was just another notch on my XL belt – I added his praises of my body and his romantic interest in me to my arsenal of retorts against the bitch in my head, and went on

with my life, fully intending to gather more notches along
the way.

12

London, UK, May 2006

The basement common room of the University College London dorm is nearly deserted, which is just as well because we're a pretty big crowd. Not to mention loud, which I guess is to be expected when you take ten American students studying abroad in Brighton, give them free train tickets into London for the weekend in the name of 'culture', and reunite them with their sorority sisters from across the pond who are studying at UCL for the semester.

I look around. Kelsey is half drunk already, her enormous boobs looking less than secure in her low-cut, embellished top. Her blonde curls brush against the faces of her two best friends and 'sisters', both of whom are currently studying at UCL, and also well on their way to being plastered. I walk over to Nik and pull up a stool. He gives me the raised eyebrows; he's the only person I knew from Wash U before I came to the UK, and he's familiar enough with my social anxiety to understand how this scene makes me feel: like I'm the fattest and least 'cool' girl in the room, and everyone can tell. He can tell I'm wishing I were a pillbug or an armadillo, anything that can roll up into itself and hide from imagined prying eyes.

Nobody else knows that, though. I've taken great pains to mask my nerves in a costume of false confidence: a friend's black tank top, tight and low-cut, printed with apples; makeup expertly applied; hair straightened into submission; and my latest boost, an *extremely* short black bubble skirt with a soft elastic waistband, which I bought from H&M to wear on nights when I want to pretend I either don't have or don't care that I have disgusting, cellulite-riddled thighs.

The costume is working so far, despite the fact that the high stool I'm sitting on makes me even more aware of my bare (and hefty) limbs. *At least I've lost a bit of weight since I've been in England – maybe my legs don't look as bad as I think.* I take a deep breath, tuck my legs as far under me as they'll go, and try to calm my heart, which is racing so fast I feel like a terrified rabbit. *Oh, who am I kidding? I may be a bit smaller than I was when I left the States, but I'm still bigger than everyone else in this room.* Despite my romantic success – or, as I now think of it, luck – in Rome, and the small gain in confidence I got from travelling alone for the rest of my Easter break, now that I'm back in England the self-consciousness is rushing back at me. Part of me wishes I'd just stayed back in the hotel room in my pajama pants, instead of pretending I could get away with trying to look hot and being social with a big group of sorority girls who intimidate the crap out of me. But it's too late to turn back now – people are starting to pull up chairs and stools, creating a kind of oval. I feel like we're about to start an intervention, but then I feel a thump on my back.

'Anne!' Kelsey is hanging on my shoulders from behind. I hold my torso straight, afraid of belly rolls. 'Are you having fun?!'

'Yeah! Sure! I mean, we only just got here, but sure.' I grin more widely than I would if it were just the two of us, but if Kelsey notices my falseness she doesn't say. 'What's next? Are we going out?'

'No, not yet. Here.' She shoves her drink into my hand. We're supposed to be pre-gaming, getting as drunk as possible on cheap 'Vodka-brand' vodka and juice before heading out to the overpriced bars. I take a big gulp and immediately regret it. My throat burns, my eyes water, and my stomach turns. It hasn't been long since Rome, when I was so hungover I wanted to die, and thought I might. *Last time I let Kelsey get me drunk. Ever.*

I grimace at her and hand her drink back – I'm just glad I haven't eaten anything recently so there's nothing in my little stomach to throw up. She grins and shrugs; she knows my feelings about alcohol lately, but I guess she figured it was worth a try. She plops down next to her two friends.

'Oh! I know!' Kelsey looks like she's just invented teleportation. 'Let's play "ten fingers" until we're drunk enough to go out! It'll help everybody get to know everybody!'

Uuuuuugh. Please hate this idea, people. I look at the unfamiliar faces, then at Nik. He looks hesitant, but everyone else is starting to get into it, so he shrugs and gives me a wicked smile.

'I'm in if you are.'

I sigh.

'Fine. It's not like I have anything embarrassing for people to find out.' *Except that whole no-experience-whatsoever thing.* I say a quick thank-you to God for Becca; at least she gave me a *little* street cred.

We all put up our hands with the fingers spread out. One of the UCL students, a guy, starts us off.

'Never have I ever . . . erm . . . had a threesome.'

It's a pretty basic start, and nobody puts down a finger. OK, so I'm not in super-kinky territory. I start to relax a bit. Jay, a socially awkward tag-along from our Brighton group, is next.

'Never have I ever had a one-night stand.' He looks proud. I'm just as pleased to be able to put a finger down with all the cool people. But then I put it back up. Then crook it, halfway.

'Wait, clarification. Full sex or just hooking up?' I turn red as I speak, but I'm also pleased to have set myself up as not *too* slutty, but not lame enough to be totally prudish.

Jay looks shocked. 'Either!'

I shrug and curl the finger into my palm.

We go around the room and my fingers stay up: cheated on a boyfriend, slept with a friend's girlfriend, had sex in a public place. Most of the other kids have one or two fingers down, except Jay, whose hands remain intact. I still only have the one down. Until we get to Kelsey.

'Never have I ever . . . um,' she looks at me with a devilish glint in her eye, 'done *more than kiss* anyone who was still in high school when I was in college!'

'You suck.' I pretend pout, and put my second finger down. One of Kelsey's friends turns to me, laughing.

'Wait, like, recently?'

'Um . . . kinda.' I crinkle my nose with affected shame.

'Ha! Try last month!' Kelsey is enjoying this way too much.

'Okaaaaay! We don't need to go there. Let's just move on. Who's next?'

As the next girl makes 'um' and 'er' noises, trying to think of something good to say, I focus on breathing in and out and try to think of my own 'never' that won't come off as too nerdy. *Never have I ever had a serious boyfriend. Slept with more than one guy. Been the hottie that every guy wants to get with. Had two guys fight over me. Felt like one of those universally acknowledged 'sexy' girls.*

'What's going on? And more importantly, can I play?' The confident voice carries from the doorway, sliding easily on a posh British accent.

'Shane!' Kelsey's friends jump up to hug the interloper, a young guy who instantly catches my attention. He looks like a Beatle – longish, effortless hair, rectangular-framed glasses, skinny tie, schoolboy blazer with some sort of cheeky badge advertising some band I'm way too lame to have heard of. I adjust my position on the stool, tucking flab and sucking in my stomach. It's the first time tonight I've felt like flirting. But Shane is already swarmed with girls – even Kelsey and her friends have leapt up to introduce themselves. I stay put. *It's never gonna happen anyway.*

Shane's arrival has spared me my turn at ten fingers. He's heading off to a bar in Angel and he's invited the lot of us, so we gather our things and everyone but me chugs their drink. Outside, the night is cool but soft, a perfect summer evening. I hang back from the group, sticking close to Nik while the girls cluster up ahead. On the bus to Angel, I hold onto the most isolated post I can find – Shane keeps looking at me, and it's making me nervous. I'm terrified he'll realise I think he's cute, and I don't have the energy to muster the faux confidence to put myself out there tonight, so I just flash him a polite smile and then stare out the window in what I hope looks like a disinterested manner.

The bar is loud, and dark, but not too crowded. We order drinks – I get a screwdriver, and then try to avoid tasting or smelling it all night – and break into small groups to perform our version of mingling. I stand on the edge of a circle and listen to Kelsey and her friends tell stories about their mutual 'sisters'; Nik and I hover awkwardly together, trying to think of something to say; Kelsey flirts with a guy at the bar and I play wing woman. And then, before I really realise what's happening, I'm alone at the window with Shane.

We chatter about random things for a bit – where I'm from, what he's studying, how he knows the other Wash U girls – and then his face is really close to mine. He smells like aftershave and alcohol. I don't pull away, but I also don't quite comprehend what's going on until his tongue is in my mouth.

I'm startled, and think of breaking away, but then his hand is on my lower back, pulling me to him, and I start to go all tingly. *Holy shit, this guy is really good.* I return the kiss, hesitantly at first, then harder, and before I have a minute to think we're full-on making out in front of everyone in the bar.

He's everywhere: hands on my ass, mouth on my neck, hair in my face. It's *hot*, hot enough that I even forget to wonder if his groping is pulling my skirt up and showing my pale, jiggly ass to the entire bar. I'm beginning to think I could do this all night, when Jay, who has apparently been standing next to us this whole time, throws up on the floor, and some of it splatters onto my bare toes.

*

When I told my friends at home about that night in London with the Beatles kid, they all asked the same question: 'Oh my God, how drunk *were* you?' It wasn't such a ridiculous thing to ask; I was probably the least experienced twenty-one-year-old they all knew, and yet here I was, in the space of a month, hooking up with two different complete strangers – British strangers, no less! It was pretty nuts.

But that was what I loved about it. My time in Brighton had been a completely new experience for me, filled with sorority girls and dorm-kitchen drink-offs and alcohol-fuelled clubbing that lasted into the wee small hours and ended with terrible fast food served by a guy who was so high he frequently screwed up our orders. I lived on Strongbow and cheap tequila, hummus slathered on flour tortillas, and bites of a huge Cadbury's Fruit and Nut bar that sat on my bookshelf; the occasional inconvenient bus trip to the supermarket was followed by a 'fancy' dinner of pan-fried salmon and asparagus doused in balsamic vinegar. I was too busy adapting to my new surroundings to worry much about my diet (although I was certainly careful not to overdo it on sweets or fatty foods, since I shared a bathroom with the rest of my hallmates), and luckily my weight seemed pretty stable so I didn't have to worry about that either, beyond the usual constant concern about being the biggest girl in the room. For the first time in my life, I was living completely on my own, in a single room, cooking for myself without the backup of a food hall nearby, and throwing myself head-long into new social situations with people I would never have spent time with at Wash U – people who got drunk regularly, who knocked on my door and handed me a bottle of cheap red wine with a straw stuck in it and ordered me to get ready for the clubs, who made out with random boys and didn't worry about what that meant. It was crazy, and new, and fun, and I let myself jump in with both feet. Of course, I often had to fake the enthusiasm, because I wasn't close enough to anyone in Brighton to indulge my depression or self-hatred. Nobody would understand what I was going through, so even on days when I woke up despising myself, I had to either hide myself in my room until it passed (which I did, some days) or pretend everything was OK. I learned a new phrase: 'Fake it 'til you make it' – and I did, I faked it like a champ. My reward was two new hook-ups and a few months of feeling like a normal person, even if eighty per cent of my actions were based on completely false confidence.

When we got back to the hotel that night in London – after I scrubbed my feet furiously under scalding water in the bar bathroom and then went back to meet my friends, who'd been kicked out – one of Kelsey's friends turned and looked at me with respect in her eyes. 'You looked like a really good kisser,' she said, and I laughed.

'What does that mean? How can I *look* like a good kisser?'

She shrugged. 'You just did. It was hot.' This girl had a big mouth, with a tongue stud, and when she said 'hot' she looked a bit like a Valley Girl lizard, but I wanted her to say it over and over again, sticking out her pierced tongue and unhinging her jaw: 'haaaaawt'.

I liked her more in that moment than I ever had. And I liked both her and Kelsey immensely when they told me they also thought Shane was hot, and would have definitely made out with him if he'd tried. I was bursting with pride. Never mind that I'd been puked on, or that we'd subsequently lost Jay and Nik had to go looking for him, or that Shane had irritated the crap out of me on the way back to the hotel, holding my hand while using his other arm to knock over random barricades and throw things into the street – I saw that evening through a haze of bliss. I couldn't stop grinning; I'd just made out with a guy that *other girls liked too, and holy shitballs he chose ME.*

I'd never in my life felt like the most desirable girl in the room. Even the month before, when Guy went after me so fervently, I'd convinced myself that he was merely low on options (Kelsey had already set her sights on Tom). But that night in London, there were some good-looking single girls in our group, and even more in the bar. I avoided Shane as best I could, and still he sought me out. And, amazingly, I felt no need whatsoever to analyse *why*. It didn't matter why – he went after me, and he was a great kisser, and I had fun and felt desirable, and that was really all I cared about. The beauty of a city the size of London was that I would likely never see him again, so even if he *had* done it out of some perverse desire to humiliate me, I would never have to know. And somehow, maybe because of the chemistry we had, I didn't think his motives were so cruel.

Maybe the best thing about that night with Shane was that I got exactly what I wanted, and what I hadn't dared go for: I got a one-night hook-up, without so much as a 'Let's keep in touch' at the end. Shane had merely walked me to my hotel, kissed me quickly on the lips, and said goodbye. And I was thrilled, not least because things *hadn't* been so clear with Guy, who was intending to visit me in Brighton the following weekend. I tried not to think about that, though, because it just made me feel guilty, as if I'd somehow *betrayed* this random penpal of mine. So instead I focused on reliving the evening: the sensation of his lips on my throat; the image of the entire group of students staring at us when we finally came up for air; the way he kept whispering 'You're so hot' against my skin.

That night, after we had brushed our teeth and gotten into our pajamas, I slipped into my single bed and lay awake, grinning. Kelsey and the girls had spent the past hour laughing at my excitement, but their gentle mockery hadn't dulled it at all. *He picked me. He picked ME*. The words ran through my mind like silk, luxurious but slippery; behind the pleasure was fear, that I would wake up in the morning and discover I'd made it all up, or, worse, it had happened but he was gross. My only consolation on that front was that I'd been stone-cold sober all day, which was more than I could say for the rest of them.

I barely slept that night, what with all the adrenalin running through my blood. The next day, we headed back to Brighton on the train, loaded down with haphazardly packed bags and hot cups of coffee. I was the only one who wasn't hungover. Once we settled in, my poor friends leaned their heads on windowpanes and each other's shoulders and tried to sleep, while I sat in the aisle and watched the green hills roll by, thinking over and over again, *he picked me*.

13

Brighton, UK, May 2006

When Guy leaves my dorm room to go to the bathroom down the hall, I make my move. I shut the curtains over the single window, whip my dress off over my head, and wiggle out of my undies and bra. Without looking in the mirror, I smooth my hair and run my tongue over my teeth, then lick my fingers and drag them under my lower eyelids to catch any mascara or eyeliner that's drifted off my lashes during the day. I'm starting to get nervous now – he could come back any minute – so to keep from bailing on the plan I focus on readying every body part now on display, which is all of them.

I sniff under my arms; I smell OK, but the run down to meet Guy at the bus stop has made the cucumber and melon fragrance of my deodorant less noticeable, and I know how much he likes it. I pull the plastic cap off and give my armpits a quick swipe.

Finally, I find the bow in my desk drawer. I bought it at Paperchase last week, when Guy told me he was definitely coming to visit. It's one of those classic cheesy gift bows:

shiny paper ribbon, looped a hundred times until it makes a rounded star shape. This one is green, and big – about the size of half an orange. I peel the backing off the square sticker-paper and bring the bow closer to my body, but then I hesitate. *Where do I put this damn thing?*

I hover the bow over my right breast, then my left. *Too off-centre.* I move it down farther, to my nakedest body part. *Too obvious!* I shift it from place to place – hip (*too much cellulite*), forehead (*too weird!*), throat (*too much like an awkward pendant*) – and finally settle on my chest, just below my collarbone on the left-hand side. I press the sticky corners to my skin and look down at myself.

What the hell am I doing?

For a split second, I consider ripping the bow off, chucking it in the trash, and putting on my fluffy robe. But then I think about Guy's face whenever I take off my clothes in front of him – the admiration in his eyes, the way his hands seem almost afraid to touch me – and I can't help smiling. *I bet I look ridiculous*, I think, but I laugh a little anyway.

I hear a movement in the hall, and my breath catches in my throat. I position myself behind the door and immediately start to panic. I put my hands over my breasts – *No, that'll just make them go all warm and soft and saggy* – I move them to my thighs – *too posed* – my hips – *too sassy* – and then finally settle them gently over my stomach. I try to breathe normally. My upper lip is sweating a little bit, so I wipe it off with a finger and then bring the hand back down into position.

Guy knocks and calls out, 'It's me.'

'Come in.' I try to sound neither nervous nor faux-seductive. It's harder than I thought it would be.

The door swings open and Guy peers around it. I back a little further into the corner so he can't see me right away.

'Anne?' He turns around and there I am, naked but for a bow and an awkward smile. Blushing madly.

Guy's jaw drops, and for a terrible second I'm sure he's as disgusted as he should be. *I should never have done this. Holy shit, what ever made me think I was anywhere near sexy enough to pull this off?* But then he steps toward me with his arms out, and smiles. I can't tell whether he's turned on or amused, but either one is better than grossed out. I laugh at myself, suddenly comfortable in my own silliness.

'What's this for?'

'Well, you're a big high-school graduate now.' I cringe, even as I smile. 'What's a cougar to do but reward all your hard work with a present?'

He grins. One hand fingers the loops on the bow, while the other hand wraps around my lower back and pulls me into him. *Well, at least now I know he's turned on!*

'This is the best graduation gift any guy could ask for,' he says, his voice deep, and muffled by his face in my neck. 'Now, do I get to unwrap you or what?'

He peels the bow off my chest slowly, careful not to hurt me, and pushes me back onto the bed. I tilt my head toward the door behind him.

'Lock it.'

*

An hour later, I lie on my side with Guy wrapped around me

from behind, his strong, hairy chest pressed against my back, his rough hands gently stroking my arm. I rest my head back against him and close my eyes.

'Wow.'

Guy is kissing my shoulders, and I feel his lips curl into a smile against my skin.

'Yeah? I thought so.'

I carefully shift my body on the narrow single bed, twisting in his arms to look up at his face.

'I mean ... Jesus Christ.' I laugh quietly. 'I'm not gonna lie, after what happened in Rome, I wasn't sure what to expect, but ... just, *wow.*'

Guy blushes and furrows his brow.

'Hey, I was very drunk in Rome, and I was nervous as hell, so it's not like I was on top form.'

I shake my head. The last thing I want is for him to think I'm insulting him.

'No, I know, it's just, well, guys say that all the time, don't they? "I was drunk." And usually, from what I hear at least, it doesn't really mean anything. I mean, it does, in terms of, er, *firmness*, but in terms of overall performance ...' *Nice, Anne. Way to ruin the moment.* I scramble for a recovery. 'Basically, you rocked my world just now. Just take the compliment.'

Guy grins and ducks his head in acknowledgement. 'Well, what can I say? I just love this body.' His hand glides down my arm and then over my hip and my bent leg to my knee. 'I want to ravish you every second.'

I open my mouth to protest – *How can that possibly be true? If the light were on he'd see all sorts of disgustingness, and his hand is sliding over a hot mess of cellulite right now* – but he leans down to kiss me before I can get a word out.

'If you don't believe me,' he whispers when our lips part, 'maybe you'll believe this.' He presses himself against me and my eyes widen.

'Already?'

He starts kissing my neck and I feel myself melt into him.

'I guess there *is* something to be said for younger guys . . .'

'Shhh,' he mutters into my skin. His mouth moves down my body and mine finally falls silent.

*

We had sex six times that night. We might have done it more but the last condom in my Wash U student health centre baggie was some weird Japanese brand that was way too tight. And thank God for that – as it was I walked like John Wayne for days after Guy left, ambling down the side-walk wincing and grinning at the same time.

By the time I'd gotten back to UK soil after my Easter holiday in Europe, Guy and I had started emailing multiple times a day, and he'd begun to talk about visiting me. He'd also started to sound like a boyfriend again, signing his emails with 'lots of love' and talking about the two of us in the future tense. I was terrified, not just of the speed with which he seemed to be getting attached, but also of my own feelings. I responded by freaking out to my friends about how this crazy kid was acting like he was in love with me, what a freak, etc., etc. (I also responded by hooking up with someone else.) Which meant that a month later, when Guy skipped Saturday class to make the six-hour, two-bus trip from Gloucestershire to come visit me for one night in Brighton, he didn't get the warmest reception from all of my friends.

But he certainly got a welcome from me. Out the window went my resolve to stay detached and my insistence that he sleep on the floor of my single room. Within two hours of his arrival at the bus station – an event for which I'd dressed up, arrived twenty minutes early, and been so flustered with nerves that I left a £20 note on the table of the cafe where I waited – we were strolling through the lanes like old lovers. We shared a pizza and made googly eyes at each other between bites of banoffee pie; we lay in the park in the sun, my head on his chest, just breathing each other in; we spent the entire night together in bed, talking and kissing and, yes, having sex.

It was mind-blowing. Not just the sex (or finding out how well endowed he was – how had I missed *that* in Rome?), but also the shift in the way my world worked: all of a sudden, here was this other body that was mine to touch and hug and hold as I pleased. I'd expected Guy to be a resource for my own feelings about *my* body – another external source to balance out my own self-hatred, and a useful distraction from my obsession with my ugliness – but I didn't plan on being so interested in *his*. The physical comfort we shared was something I'd never really experienced before, even as I'd revelled in the joys of hand-holding with Josiah. This was different. And the emotional comfort was different too. Because Guy was so sappy and silly, I didn't feel like I needed to be cool and disinterested. I didn't need to pretend I was more experienced than I was, or act like I didn't care whether he hooked up with other girls. In fact, that very weekend we agreed to be exclusive. Exclusive! We'd known each other a month, had been in the same room for three days out of that month, and lived an eight-hour bus ride apart. Not to mention that I was headed back to America in two months, there was a three-year age gap between us, and oh by the way he was still in high school.

But that was what Guy did to me: he made me forget all my reasons *not* to do things. I forgot that I shouldn't eat banoffee pie in front of him, because he was enjoying it as much as I was and his hands seemed to love my ample hips. I forgot that he was too young for me because I was the one telling fart jokes while he quoted *The Waste Land* with relish. I forgot that our pairing was completely illogical and logistically difficult because it felt so easy to be with him. I even managed to forget sometimes that I hated my body – I could be completely down on myself when he wasn't around, and then the minute he showed up and wrapped his arms around me I'd feel small and girly again. Everything just worked when we were together, and because I figured we wouldn't be together once I left the UK I wanted to have a good time while it lasted. And boy did I fulfil that desire.

May and June were a flurry of sex-filled weekends. He visited me when he could, and I visited him twice in Cheltenham (we had to get a B&B room and watch our backs in town, because he was *hiding me from his mum*. Oh, the shame). We spent hours just lying in bed saying alternately dirty and mushy things to each other. It was a whole new experience for me, and I was loving every minute.

Josiah had taught me that sex could be a liberating force in my fight against my insecurities. Becca had shown me how to use my body to my advantage, how to *seduce* those few odd folk who found me attractive. Both of them had added to the voices for the opposition, slightly minimising the importance I gave to the voice of my own self-hatred. But it wasn't until Guy came along that I understood just how much having a legitimate, longer-term sex life would change the way I viewed myself, and my body.

I became a different person when sex was involved. I did things I would never have even thought of doing in the past. I had sex in a hotel lobby bathroom, and we weren't even staying there – we had to pause the action right at the good part while someone came in, peed, and washed her hands. When Guy came out to San Francisco to visit me for three weeks once I'd left Brighton, I spent a weekend with him at a romantic hotel up the coast and we barely left the room or even got dressed – we had sex twenty-three times in one day, no lie. I even had sex in a train bathroom, propped up on the teeny sink basin – well, OK, I didn't put all my weight on it because I was afraid to break it, and I failed to completely forget that we were in a *stinky train bathroom*, but hey, I still did it.

In the space of a summer I went from a barely experienced girl who wanted nothing more than a little hand-holding and maybe a nice quiet orgasm in the evening-time (after dinner and a movie of course), to a wild and crazy cougar-lady who was desperate to satisfy her insatiable younger man by whatever means necessary. It was a bit of a jolt, but it was also addictive, and so I agreed to date him long-distance, despite the voice in my head screaming that long-distance relationships never worked. I shrugged off my concerns; better to have crazy-good sex and snuggles a few times a year and to pine the rest of the time, I figured, than to have none of those things, *all* the time. Besides, when we weren't in the same country, we could still communicate via email and phone, and I was unwilling to lose the person who had become my biggest emotional and physical support in the fight against my insecurities – simply by *existing* as a presence in my life, Guy made me feel better about myself. He never didn't want me or thought I looked ugly or fat, and even as I told myself that his view of me was skewed or tempered somehow – that he saw me through rose-tinted sex goggles – and tortured myself and him with my attempts to 'figure him out', I couldn't deny that I loved how he made me feel.

Besides, I had to admit that Guy wasn't just good for my body image – he was good for my body (which was, in turn, good for my body image). I'd had a feeling I was losing weight since we'd started dating, but I didn't have a set of scales in Brighton – and besides, once I met Guy I was too happy to be obsessively weighing myself any more (Guy loved my body so much I almost stopped caring what anyone else thought, including me). Once I got back to the States, though, my bathroom scales confirmed what I'd suspected: I'd lost weight while I was in Brighton, and I could tell from the way my clothes fit that I'd lost the majority of it toward the end of the trip (post-Guy). I was down to 175 pounds, lighter than I'd been since right after the surgery, when I'd dipped down briefly and then returned to 185. And I hadn't even been trying to lose weight, that was the beauty of it – I'd heard my friends complain about gaining weight when they got a new boyfriend, because they were going out to restaurants more often and spending a lot of time cuddling on the couch, but my new boyfriend had made me thinner! I was elated, and when I told Guy he laughed and said he reckoned it was all the 'activity' I'd been doing, on top of that activity taking away my time for snacks. We started calling it Guy's sex diet – all I knew was, it was the only diet I'd ever *wanted* to stay on.

So we gave the long-distance thing a shot, and it actually worked pretty well. During my final year at college, back in St Louis, we spent far too many hours on the phone, moping about how much we missed each other, and when Guy was able to visit we more than made up for lost time. It was the same whirlwind, fling-like fun we'd had in the UK, an extension of the sex-prioritising 'honeymoon phase' that went on for much longer than it probably would have, had we been living in the same country. Even after we'd been dating for about a year and we'd cooled down a little, Guy's attitude toward me didn't change. He still seemed to find me totally irresistible, and I still didn't get it. But the difference after that first year was that I no longer felt such a need to get it – most of the time I just appreciated it.

I'd worried for a long time that he would one day realise how utterly undesirable I was, but he didn't. And all that time, while I was doing everything I'd ever wanted to do before I'd had the opportunity (and anything he wanted to do lest he up and leave me), something amazing was happening: an intense intimacy had started to spring up between us. And I don't just mean the physical intimacy that inevitably comes out of repeated sexual encounters – I mean something deeper, something more essential to changing my attitude about myself and relationships. It was an intimacy created not just by the good times, but by the awkward times: the spinal cracks and muscle spasms that resulted from overzealous foreplay; those panicked moments of 'no no not THERE'; the little puff of air that escaped from my body while we were entwined in a tender post-coital embrace and caused me to lock myself in the bathroom for twenty minutes while Guy suffocated with laughter in the hall. All those things would have caused me to die from shame in earlier years – oh, the humiliating unfeminine-ness of it! But with Guy, I didn't feel like I had to be perfect in every other way in order to make up for the stark imperfection of my body; Guy thought my body *was* perfect (as mad as he must have been to think so), and those little slip-ups and embarrassing accidents were nothing more than entertaining stories, in his mind.

Those were the moments when I knew – really understood, with more certainty than I knew anything else – that here was a guy I could really trust. I'd gotten a hint of it early on, that first night in Brighton after we'd had sex for the first time. I was sitting on the bed, completely naked and surprisingly OK with that fact, and Guy was crouched in front of me on the floor. He gently took my hands, turned my palms upward, and slid his fingers lightly up my body until they were skimming over the red, ropey scars on the insides of my upper arms. I stiffened a bit, but I didn't stop him. His gaze wandered over the skin for a while, taking in the freshness and length of the scars, and then he looked up, into my eyes, and asked, 'What happened to you?' I wasn't sure what to do – I barely knew him, really, and I hadn't planned on getting into my messy life story so early on, but at the same time I felt closer to him than I'd ever felt to any other guy. I bit the bullet.

'Do you really want to know? It's a long story and kind of personal, but I'll tell you if you don't think it'll make you feel awkward.'

He nodded. He seemed sincere, so I told him.

'When I was seventeen I had weight-loss surgery, that's what these little scars are from,' I pointed to the two short, faded marks on the middle of my stomach, 'and then when I lost a hundred pounds I had all this ... leftover skin ...' I tried not to shudder. 'And so I had it removed from my arms and stomach,' I gestured to the scar across my lower belly, 'and hopefully I can do the legs soon.' I breathe in and out. *That actually wasn't so long after all.*

My heart pounded as I began to worry. Maybe I'd shared too much too soon; would he decide now that I really wasn't kidding about carrying a lot of baggage, and I was right to tell him I wasn't worth his time? If he did think about any of those things, he didn't say. He just kissed the ends of my scars, on the insides of my elbows, then he stood, kissed my forehead, and said, 'Thank you for telling me.' He sat down next to me on the bed and we snuggled up and watched a cheesy American comedy on my laptop, and my heart soothed itself.

After that, I only felt closer to Guy. I knew I could trust him with my body, which he treated like it belonged to a supermodel instead of a pear-shaped post-GB mess, and because I could trust him with my body I understood that I could trust him with my heart as well, because as much as my body and my mind are so often at odds, they're also inextricably linked and bonded.

Guy's insatiability eventually became overwhelming for me, and we had to tone it down, but in that first year it was just what I needed – it was probably the only way he could have broken down the walls I'd spent so many years building up, convincing myself that I wasn't attractive in and of myself, that I could never hold a man's attention and any man who momentarily lapsed in concentration and hooked up with me would eventually come to his senses. Guy never seemed to lose interest, even for a day, and most importantly his constant need for me was just that: for *me*. He wasn't satisfied with anything else, whether it was porn or masturbation or even my frustrated suggestion that he go find some skinny chick to pick up at a party (because of course, even if he didn't, *I* always had to bring thinness into the equation). It was irritating sometimes to be the only answer to his desire, but it was also exceedingly validating – especially as toning down the sex and going out to eat together meant I'd gained back the fifteen or twenty pounds I lost when we were first dating! So even as I was complaining about feeling pressured or begging him to just get off and leave me alone to *read a goddamn book*, I was always conscious of how unusual this man was, and how lucky/random it was that *I'd* been the one to find him. I mean, what normal man fantasises only about his pudgy partner, looking at porn only under duress and pressure from his girlfriend?

It took time, and work, and a *lot* of exasperating conversations and arguments, but when we got past the issues caused by Guy's libido, what we were left with was an extremely close bond. There was nobody in the world I trusted more than Guy: he was the first person I wanted to talk to or see when something notable happened in my life, good or bad; he was the only person I'd ever wanted to go to sleep with every night and wake up to every morning; I missed him when he was sitting right next to me, sucked into the computer (of course the minute he turned to pay attention to me I shushed him and went back to my book). Oh, and the other thing we were left with? An awesome sex life, full of experimentation and laughter and mutual desire and love. Which was something I'd never allowed myself to hope for from life.

When I was a virgin and wishing desperately not to be, I used to fantasise about having someone to have sex with, but that was all I wanted: sex. I wasn't thinking as far as intimacy or experimentation or even orgasms (I could do those myself, thank you very much). When I was finally introduced to the world of sex, after a long wait outside in the rain, I got just what I was expecting: normal, OK, missionary sex with someone I figured was probably a decent person and who was capable of giving me a mediocre orgasm. It was more than I'd ever been given, and it was plenty. I planned on my sex life being basically the same for the rest of my life – a little better here, a little worse there. As long as the guy wasn't an asshole or a premature ejaculator, I figured, I was doing pretty well. I'd even been pleasantly surprised to discover that, rather than sex being something I had to work to suppress my body issues in order to enjoy, it was actually something that could help me escape them entirely, if only for a brief time.

But with Guy, I got so much more than I'd bargained for. Not only did I find someone who was willing – even raring – to have sex with my yucky body on a regular basis, but he also turned out to have magic hands, in more ways than one. When Guy touched me, I felt like a completely different person; if I closed my eyes and focused on the sensation, I could almost imagine that his hand was running over a firm, curvaceous butt, instead of the puddle of flesh that I saw when I allowed myself to look over my shoulder. He was an illusionist, a hypnotist, and under his spell I felt attractive, even *sexy*. There were moments during sex with Guy that I felt like a sex goddess, a slinky little minx – it was almost an out-of-body experience, except that it had everything to do with the body, *my* body, and for once that was a good thing. As for the sex itself, I'd really had no idea what I was in for with Guy. The night we met, he practically maimed me. He licked my face and tormented my downstairs, but for some reason I still liked him. So I let him try again, and boy was I ever glad I did. Who knew that this random eighteen-year-old from a private boys' school in Bumfuck Spa, England, would have any idea what he was doing? Even if we hadn't gotten close – if he hadn't broken down my defences and wormed his way so deep into my heart that I had no idea who I ever was before I met him – it still would have been worth giving him a second chance just for the sex.

That first night in Rome, sex was all I was looking for. I wanted a one-night stand; I was lonely, and kind of horny, and on a travel high. I got drunk, met a boy, and did inappropriate things with him all over the city. It was supposed to be a bit of fun – something I'd never done before, and something that had always scared me. When I woke up the next morning and looked over at him, I felt the terror rush back; I spent the next two days waiting for him to burst out laughing and show me the YouTube video he'd posted of me under the title 'Fat chick thinks she's hot'. For months after that first email, I kept waiting for him to shout *PSYCH!* and run off into the slender arms of someone better-looking, the two of them laughing at my naïveté. 'A great figure?' they would snort. 'Her?'

Not only did that never happen, but it almost seemed as if every day he was *more* excited to be dating me. And after a couple of years with him, I somehow stopped waiting for the day Guy would snap out of his delusion and realise I was disgusting. I stopped telling myself to hold back my own feelings, just a little, to protect myself from the day that he would recognise his mistake, and I finally allowed myself to see the relationship as more than just 'a learning experience', as something that could really be for keeps. Delusional or not, Guy woke up in the morning and looked at me, at my smeared mascara and frizzy hair, and smiled. Every day. And when we walked into parties or restaurants, when I pulled away from him a bit in hopes of sparing his reputation, his arm would snake around my waist and pull me close.

Even though I still struggled with feelings of disgust and misery about my body, I was beginning to wonder whether what I saw in the mirror was really representative of what other people saw; if Guy could love my body so much, surely it couldn't possibly be as revolting as I thought it was? I loved Guy, and I trusted him, but I had also spent the past fifteen years in absolute certainty that my body was unattractive, so I was confused as to whom to believe. But what if neither of us was entirely right or wrong? Maybe my 'real' body lay somewhere between the monster in my nightmares and the girl of his dreams.

Consistency is key, isn't that what they say? Well, after a couple of years of consistent affection and attention and desire, for me and *for* my body, rather than in spite of it (which was all I'd ever dared to hope for), I began to think Guy might just be making an impression on me. I even began to believe that maybe, after a few more years, I'd start to see more than just glimpses of the beautiful woman he was so proud to be sleeping with – maybe, through Guy loving me, I could finally learn to love me too.

III

THE AFTERMATH

14

London, October 2007

I pull the canvas skirt over my butt, stuff my hips in under the waistband, and button the first few snaps that run up the front of the blue patterned fabric. I fasten the safety pin where the material gapes open, right over my crotch, and suck in my breath to get the top three snaps. The tank top I picked out earlier is lying on the unmade bed; it's one of my favourites, a racerback style with green and black curlicues on it that look like snails. I lean across the chest at the foot of the bed, grab the tank, and put it on, pulling and stretching the cheap cotton so it sits just right and covers all the little bits of flesh that are doing their damnedest to poke out of the top of my skirt. And then I make my first mistake: I look in the mirror.

When Guy comes into the bedroom five minutes later, the small expanse of floor is strewn with clothes. He has to push to get the door all the way open, because it gets stuck on a pair of inside-out Bermuda shorts. The skirt I used to love so much has been relegated to dustbunny duty, shoved under the dresser so I won't have to look at it any more. The tank top that once made me feel so confident and curvy is inside out, squashed into a ball and hurled into the farthest corner I can find in our tiny London flat. Three or four more outfits, tried on in an attempt to cling to the last shards of my sanity, litter the floor around my bare feet.

I look up as the door opens, and Guy's face says it all: *You look a total fright*. My mascara is probably running all over my face – the tears started around outfit number three – and I know my hair is frizzing and my face red from the body heat I've got going in my frenzy. *I should just stop this nonsense and put on some fucking clothes.* But I can't.

'Anne, what on earth?' Guy steps past the dresser and around the bed, coming towards me with his arms out, ready to hug my insanity out of me. But I leap outside his reach.

'Don't! Just *don't* touch me.' I try to breathe normally but my heart is racing. I feel wound, sprung, as if in order to survive I need to explode out of my skin in every direction. I shift my weight quickly between my feet, back and forth, my hands shaking. Guy's eyes widen.

'OK, OK,' his palms go up as he takes a step back, almost bumping into the full-length mirror that started it all, which is leant up against the wall by the dresser. 'Why don't you just tell me what's happening and we'll sort it out.'

I hate how calm he sounds. I want to hit him, but instead I just shout.

'What's happening is I don't have any CLOTHES because I'm too FAT FOR EVERYTHING and I know we have this thing and we need to leave in five minutes but I CAN'T GO OUT THERE BECAUSE I'M A

MONSTER.' As I say this last part, I start sobbing again, and fidgeting even more. I pace back and forth in the tiny space between the foot of the bed and the front windows, desperate to go anywhere, be anywhere but inside my own skin.

'Look,' Guy is approaching me again, but I give him a wild-eyed stare and he backs off, 'look, what if I just pick something and you put it on and then we go, and you don't look in the mirror, we just go. Would that work, do you think?'

I'm hiccoughing, and I try again to breathe but my lungs are shuddering and my nose is running. I shrug, as if maybe his idea could work. *It won't work. It won't make me thinner. I'll still be disgusting and huge and rolling out of whatever he gives me to wear.*

Guy scans the room. As he turns to glance behind him, he spots the edge of blue patterned canvas peeking out from under the dresser, and he bends down to retrieve it.

'I thought you wanted to wear this today. You looked so lovely in it last weekend –'

I rip the skirt from his hands as he tries to dust it off, and throw it back on the floor.

'No, I couldn't have, unless I've gained like thirty pounds since then, because I look *hideous* in it now! I put it on and my fat spilled out and it's too short and I hate my fat legs that the surgery didn't fix and I hate my knock knees and my stupid fat cellulitey skin! I HATE IT.'

I'm starting to hyperventilate now, I can feel my chest tightening. I back away from Guy's reach again, but I bump up against the windowsill and he catches me and holds me tight against his chest. He's warm, and strong, and normally this is exactly where I need to be when I'm losing my shit, but right now I just feel tense and my neck hurts from the way my head has to turn and his slow, steady heartbeat in my ear just makes mine race faster with fury that he can be so calm when I'm falling apart.

I shove back.

'We don't have time for this bullshit! We have to go and I have be normal in front of my friend and –' I dissolve into tears again. By now I'm barely breathing at all, and what little air I am getting is laced with asthmatic wheezing.

I try to push Guy away again, but he pulls me in tighter.

'Shh, just breathe,' he says, his hands stroking my back, 'we don't need to be on time. We don't even need to go. If you don't think you can face it, we'll just call and cancel.'

At that, the fury wells up in me and I direct it at him, again.

'We can't just CANCEL. We've been planning this lunch date for fucking MONTHS and if I cancel now I'll look like a total asshole! Why does this shit always happen when I NEED TO BE SANE? I just want to hack it all off with a cleaver!'

I've broken free of his embrace, and I'm grabbing at my flesh when I say this last part, pulling great handfuls of hip and butt away from the bone, showing him how loose and flabby and *disgusting* my body is. Wanting him to see what I hate so much, while at the same time hoping he can't. Hoping he sees only good things, even if that means one of us is totally unhinged.

Guy's face goes pale and he puts his hands on my arms, forcing me to drop myself and stand still for a second.

'Anne. Look at me, Anne.'

I can't. I look at his chin.

'Anne, don't ever do that. Please, don't let yourself talk like that. I couldn't stand to watch you hurt yourself.'

I nod, slowly, but inside all I can think is that what I do or don't tell him makes no difference. *I'll still think it. I'll still want to do it, still wish I weren't so goddamn practical and concerned about blood and scarring. I'll always think it would be endlessly satisfying to slice a chunk of flesh off my thigh and feel all this anxiety turn into physical, treatable pain.*

'Good. Now lie down.'

I obey, letting him push me onto the bed and get behind me. I claw for the covers, hating the way my hip bunches against the elastic in my underwear when I lie on my side, and for once he helps me cover up. Guy's left arm stretches under my head, and his right arm wraps around my ribs, pulling me in as tightly as he can. I'd be afraid of suffocating if I weren't already halfway there.

'Now,' he says, his voice hot in my ear, 'I know it's difficult, but I really need you to breathe. Just take it one breath at a time, following me.' He breathes in and out in exaggeratedly long, deep breaths, his chest pressing into my back when he inhales, and releasing me when he exhales. I try to follow his motions. My torso is shaking, hard, and I can only get tiny gulps of air, which I exhale in low wailing sounds.

It'll never work, I think, *I'll never breathe again. I'll never feel normal again. I may as well just let myself suffocate.* But somewhere in my mind, my logical self fights back. *Stop it. Just stop it. Just do as he says and breathe.*

I lean back into Guy's warm chest and put all my strength into the simple process of inhaling and exhaling. I try to mimic the sound of my ragged breath in my mind to keep it from focusing on the hot, sticky feeling where the flesh is folding at my waistline, or the tickle on the bridge of my nose as yet another tear slides sideways out of my right eye and into my left, or the fact that Guy's right pinky is drifting dangerously close to the pool of skin where my belly meets the bed. The only way to stop myself from thinking about those things is to think nothing at all. And the only way to do that is to copy in my mind the loudest sound in the room, my ragged breath:

Hu-hu-hu-huh whoooooooooo hu-hu-hu-huh whoooooooooo hu-hu-hu-huh whoooooooooo . . .

At some point, when my tears have dried into itchy patches of salt all over my face, when the wailing exhale I'm so focused on has gotten smoother and quieter, Guy leaves me alone to go cancel our lunch date. Without his arm around me, I curl tighter into myself, pulling my bent legs up by my chest and squeezing them until my hip muscles hurt. I bury my face in my knees, relishing the feeling of forehead on kneecap, bone on bone, savouring the pain of something hard that's a part of *my body*.

I stay like that, breathing in the smell of my skin and trying to control my shaking, for a long time. I fall asleep, and only wake up when Guy comes in to check on me. He asks if I'm OK. I manage to shake my head. I fall asleep.

*

Poor Guy. I'd bet good money that when we decided to live together, when I graduated from university with no idea what to do with my English degree and moved to London to give our long-distance love a 'real shot', Guy had no idea what he was in for. In fairness, I had no idea myself. Being with Guy had boosted my confidence more than any of the physical changes I'd made to my body; how could I predict that my body issues would come creeping back in once the initial excitement of having a boyfriend wore off, or that I would be totally overwhelmed by the change in location and feel completely out of my element in a city I thought I knew, or that the thigh lift I had right after graduation wouldn't make me feel nearly as good as the arm and stomach surgeries I'd had two years before? So I arrived in London, on a short-term work visa, with no idea what to do for a job or how to find a flat we would both like or how to live with a boyfriend without killing him over dirty dishes or a wet bathmat. And even though I was at the lower end of my weight scale, about 185 pounds, and living with someone who loved the way I looked and was proud to be seen with me, I spiralled into one of the worst periods of depression and anxiety that I'd had to deal with in over a year. I had regular freak-outs and anxiety attacks, and when I wasn't raging against my body I was laconic and self-deprecating.

I eventually got used to my surroundings – we found an apartment in Fitzrovia and I got a job as a receptionist at a dental practice in Harley Street, and London began to feel more like home. I came out of my depression a bit, and I'd like to say that really bad breakdowns happen rarely these days, but that depends on your definition of rarity. They certainly happen less often than they did in those first few months of living with Guy, and now I have long periods of relative contentment in which I don't necessarily *like* my body, but I can usually manage to bury my hatred for it, rather than feeling that dull disgust at all times. Most of the time, I can recognise the warning signs: I'll feel the depression and anger tickling at the back of my throat and I'll find a way to distract myself from my self-sabotaging mind.

Still, those calm periods are punctuated by cruel weeks of darkness in which I wake up hating myself, spend all day despairing or ranting over my disgusting form, and go to bed crying. It's not usually as dramatic as a full-blown, bedroom-destroying meltdown, but it can get pretty bad; a good year, for me, is one in which I have only one or two days where I'm so miserable and depressed and furious about my body that I have to miss school or work or a social engagement. A year entirely devoid of these occurrences is a dream I have yet to realise.

The weird thing is, I don't remember having this violent reaction to my body when I was fat. I mean, I was frustrated, and I felt helpless and sad, depressed and even desperate at times, but I don't recall anything like what I feel in my worst moments now: *fury*.

I get so angry it's scary. Not just for the few people who've seen me in this state (actually, pretty much just Guy), but for me too. I watch myself become this *beast*, feel my hands itch for some instrument with which to harm my body. I get this uncontrollable urge to manifest myself in some other body so I can go to battle with it. My soul and my body are at odds, and want nothing more than to split from each other, which is the one thing that's impossible to do.

When I was fat, I wanted to *change* my body. I tried diets, exercise, and complaining; none of it worked. But I also knew on some level that nothing slow-acting would ever work for me – I gave up too easily. And so I didn't really have a right to be mad at my body, because my mind was too much of a wuss to try hard enough to change it. And while I still felt upset that it was my lot in life to struggle with weight, I was more depressed and resigned to the world's unfairness than I was angry and self-destructive.

But that all changed when I made my first really serious effort to control my body. When I had the gastric bypass, I really thought I would finally have some power, some agency over my own hulking form. I didn't expect to look like a movie star, I just expected to be smaller, thinner, more *normal*. And when I discovered that it wasn't that easy – when I stood in front of the mirror six months after surgery comparing my naked body when I lifted the excess skin with the saggy mess when I left it hanging (*normal, gross, normal, gross*) – I was sorely disappointed.

Still, I tried to tell myself that it would be OK. I would at least have more control over my body than I had when I was obese. The playing field had been levelled, I told myself: normal people try to lose weight all the time, but the difference is they need to lose ten pounds instead of 110. Now I could be one of those normals! I could work out hard and see results within a month; I could diet and lose three pounds in a week and have it make a difference in how I looked; I could go up or down a size in clothes, and continue to shop in the same store.

I was right: the playing field *was* more level. But that didn't mean I had control. When I was fat, I didn't spend much time thinking about why I gained weight so easily – I didn't care about the gaining side of things, I just wanted to figure out how to lose. In fact, it wasn't until after I lost the initial weight that I began to wonder what caused the gaining, because now all of a sudden that was my concern: putting the weight back on. I started researching different theories of why people get fat and stay fat, and how they can lose or maintain most successfully. I became slightly obsessed with the science of weight gain – the *New York Times* website now lists every single weight-related article in the sidebar under 'Suggested for You' – but in the end, what I learned is that the science doesn't always work for *me*.

My body seems to defy rational action; diet and exercise sometimes cause me to gain weight, and often when I stop obsessing over it – if I'm on vacation or a road trip, or somewhere else where a gym and healthy food are unavailable – I'll actually lose weight. I lost fifteen pounds when I *stopped* calorie counting last year. In nine months of 1,700 calories a day (I didn't want to go too low, for fear of falling off the wagon and bingeing), with an hour and a half at the gym three days a week and yoga on my off days, I'd lost ten pounds, six of which I'd gained in the first week of the new regimen! It doesn't make sense.

And it's the senselessness that drives me mad. When I was heavier, I understood that I was more than just the victim of genetics; I knew that I also didn't try hard enough to exert control over my eating, my exercise habits, or, yes, my genetic tendency to put on weight. But because I knew I wasn't *really dedicated* to controlling my circumstances, I didn't get so angry when I couldn't control them with wishes and what-ifs and half-hearted attempts. Now, when I've spent countless amounts of time and money on a million different diet and exercise routines and had four expensive, painful surgeries, when I've spent months counting every calorie or trying not to slip in pools of sweat at bikram yoga classes, every day is a struggle not to focus on how little control I truly have over this body I'm stuck with for the rest of my life. On bad days I can get so distracted by my self-hatred that I can't even carry out a conversation with a new friend or be a supportive partner to my boyfriend. Sometimes I hear myself talking to Guy about all the crazy thoughts that go through my mind about my body, and it's like I want to shout at myself to just *shut the fuck up*. It's so bloody boring, and I'm fed up. If I can't force my body to bend to my will, I'll have to find a way to control my mind. I have to be able to get on with my life.

And sometimes I lose that battle. Sometimes all it takes is standing in front of my closet in the morning, trying to find something to wear to work. One article of clothing that won't show the bulges where the elastic in my underwear presses my soft skin, or the little dimple where my tummy-tuck scar dips in the middle, or the shelf of flesh above my butt that sticks out when I push off my back leg as I walk. On days when I can't find something to wear, as shallow as that sounds, my mind enters a dangerous territory, where every moment teeters on the verge of an outburst of self-hatred and fury followed by a period of immobility and depression.

Once I get into these moods, nothing can help bring me back for a long time. Logic, the knowledge that I can't possibly be as hideous as I think, is useless in the face of my own reflection. The loving boyfriend who can't keep his hands off my body becomes more of a reminder that my body exists (in all its foulness) than a reassurance that it's attractive. Friends and family are completely powerless against my over-active, self-sabotaging mind.

When I was heavy I often wanted to be told I wasn't fat. I hoped for reassurance, even as I knew it wouldn't be the truth. I was desperate for compliments, even as I brushed them off and denied them. I knew I was fat, but I still craved the kindness of other people's lies. Now, though, despite the fact that some sane part of me knows I'm not fat – or at least, no longer an objective definition of the term – those once-comforting words just make me angry. Guy's constant promise that he *really doesn't think I'm gross* falls on deaf ears. How can he not see what I see? How can his hands, skimming over the lumps and folds that we both know so well, not feel the revolting cellulite I feel? How can he not be as repulsed by me as I am?

Instead of fighting my own mood, I find myself fighting the rest of the world, daring them to open their eyes and *see* me, challenging Guy (and all other men) to flee from my hideous form and even more hideous emotional baggage. If a man stares at me in the street, I instantly check to make sure my bra isn't showing, or touch my teeth with my tongue to see if there's a bit of spinach lurking in there, waiting to embarrass me. When I'm in one of my dark phases, I never assume I'm stared at in a good way; every look is an assault, an accusation. *You're not one of us*, they say, looking me up and down, *you're a fraud. A big, fat fraud.*

So I've become contrary, and sometimes kind of a bitch. People say nice things to me, and I brush them off awkwardly, or if I'm a bit drunk or in a bad mood I might call them liars. I'll tell them not to insult my intelligence, or beg them not to spare my feelings, even as they protest they have no idea what I'm on about. I confuse them, because I'm confused. I have no idea what my body looks like, really; some part of me believes the other people, knows that it's my *mind* that is distorted, but I can only go with what I feel to be true, and assume that the ugly, bloated, jiggly form I grudgingly acknowledge every morning must be what they see.

One of the more ridiculous habits I've developed since the surgery is the constant comparison. Before I met Guy, I at least kept it to myself, reading trashy magazines and comparing celebrities' much-maligned 'cellulite' to the dimply mess where my thighs should be, or sitting in a coffee shop and trying to gauge the difference in depth between my tights-roll and that of my neighbour. It was mostly hidden, too, when we were long-distance, because I could pretend to be relatively normal for the short spaces of time that we were together – I was usually too busy enjoying the dates and snuggles and getting laid to talk too much about my issues, anyway – but when I graduated from college and moved to London to live with him, both of our roles changed. When I let Guy into the world in my head, I showed him how not-normal I really was, and I unwittingly signed him up as my objective observer.

We walk down the street and I watch every woman who passes. When I see one whose hips look like they might re-semble mine, or whose arms seem just a touch meatier than most, I tug Guy's arm and point the lady out. 'OK, her. Is she bigger or smaller than I am? I mean, I know her boobs are bigger, but just ignore that and look at her hip width. Sim-ilar?' He rolls his eyes, but I press on. 'I'm *serious*. This is important!'

He turns, reluctantly, and gives the woman a quick once-over. Far too quick, if you ask me – he should be studying her ass. He turns back to me with one of three looks: dis-comfort, disgust, or disinterest. Which means either: she's smaller than I am, she's much bigger than he thinks I am, or she's sort of the same, or similar enough that he feels safe brushing it off as sorted.

The problem is, I don't stop there. Once I know his re-action, I dissect the clues that I assume have led him to his judgement. Unfortunately, I often do this out loud: 'It was the hips, right? I mean, I don't think my thighs are that small, but . . .' 'Wait, so I know she's smaller but was the texture of her butt at least similar? It seemed kind of square like mine . . .' 'Oh, OK, so I'm smaller than she is, but that last woman I pointed out was about my size? But they looked the same to me!'

In general, since the surgery, I've gotten a lot more vocal about my body issues. It's strange, because I felt like they were so obvious when I was heavy, and you'd think that would make me feel comfortable addressing them out loud, but instead I was terrified of acknowledging them, of confirming people's assumptions about my self-esteem. Now, though, I bring this stuff up to people, and I'm not sure why. It's certainly not because I think I need to tell them I'm gross and fat – they can see that clearly, according to my inner bitch – but it's also not because I think my hideousness is obvious, and I need to address it. I think maybe it's just that my obsession with hating my body has grown so big I can't contain it inside me any more, and that's a problem. It consumes me, which hurts on an almost physical level, and it turns me into a bit of a monster sometimes, socially. Luckily, Guy bears the brunt of this burden patiently, allowing me to keep my friends and family just this side of so exasperated they cut me out of their lives, but I don't know how long he'll be able to be so patient.

I'm often asked whether Guy is a saint. To that I can only say: maybe. In fairness to me, he has his quirks and annoying habits, but in fairness to him, he does put up with a lot. I don't harass him about other women all that often – and I do like to defend myself by joking that at least I *encourage* him to look at other women's bodies, unlike most girlfriends

– but I can get pretty fixated at times. The thing is, I need Guy to help me translate, to help me find some common ground between what I see and hate and what the rest of the world sees and (mostly) accepts. Sometimes I worry about what I'll do if Guy and I break up; how will I ever find anyone else who's willing to liaise between me and this hostile captor of mine?

My body and I just can't seem to agree. It doesn't understand me, and I can't even begin to understand it. It responds to my attempts to change it like an unruly teenager; it won't listen, it refuses to communicate its needs in any constructive way, and it inconveniences me at every turn. But in the end, it's the only body I've got, so I have to find a way to get along with it. I can't depend on Guy to always be my judge or the answer to my consuming insecurities – not only might he leave (or, God forbid, not live longer than I do), but it's just plain unhealthy. I don't lean on him for financial support or expect him to feed and bathe me, so why do I allow myself to need his emotional support so badly?

Over the years, my perspective has changed along with my physique. The further my body has gotten from the drastic changes and physical recovery that came just after the gastric bypass, the more I've focused on it and found smaller and more specific things to nitpick. First it was the fat, then the skin. It's still the skin now, but it's also the size of the thighs and the skin that still hangs off them in certain poses, or the stretchmarks that slither like silverfish from my shoulders to my ankles, or the breasts that are more triangular than teardrop. It's always something, and it's getting exhausting.

I'm beginning to think I need to stop thinking so much.

15

Oxfordshire, UK, Christmas 2007

Oscar, who's three, and Jake, who recently turned five, are drawing and whispering in the corner of the living room. They keep darting glances at me and giggling, waiting for me to ask what they're doing – the likely result of which will be some rude crayoned image thrust in my face – but I'm no dummy. I may have only just met Guy's little brothers, but I've been around kids plenty, and I know that once you react to the noises and surreptitious glances it's all over. Best to keep your nose hidden in your book, pretending to ignore them for as long as possible, which is exactly what I'm doing.

Guy comes in to check on me and stoke the fire. Once he's poked around and caused a few satisfactory sparks, he adds another log and sits down next to me on the couch. I shift to make room for him, adjusting my clothing along the way to make sure no fleshy bits are poking out, but he ignores the extra space and leans into me. He gives me a kiss, which lingers a little too long given our audience, whom he then makes the unfortunate mistake of noticing.

The boys are watching both of us now, their earlier game forgotten in favour of this new, much more interesting prey.

'Oscar, Jake, what are you two up to?'

They dissolve into shrieks of delight and secrecy. I glare at Guy, sigh, and close my book, dog-earing the corner so I won't lose my place.

Oscar launches himself into Guy, while Jake, the more delicate of the two, tiptoes around the side of the sofa and whispers something in Guy's ear. All three boys look at me. *Fine, I'll bite.*

'What?'

Guy smiles and shoves his brothers off him. They fall to the rug, tumbling on top of each other and laughing.

'They think we're going to get married, and that I smell like poo.'

'Guy smells like POO!' The boys are rolling on the floor, so tickled by their own joke that I'm afraid we might have a mess to clean up. I ignore the marriage comment, as always, and focus instead on the part of their accusation that I know how to handle.

'Are you sure it's not *you two*?' I leap to my boyfriend's defence, though I'm not sure he deserves it – I know better than anyone that he *can* be quite stinky.

The kids stop and look at each other. Jake is red in the face.

'No!' His posh British accent sounds like 'naio'. He turns to Oscar, as if checking to see if he's been duped. Oscar does what he does best: shouts.

'It's not US. It's YOU!'

They dissolve again. Guy makes an appalled face and tries to admonish them.

'Now, boys, that's not a nice thing to say –'

I keep my calm and cut him off.

'Well, guys, I'm sorry to disappoint you, but that's simply not possible. You see, I don't do that.'

They stop giggling and stare at me, their mouths open. Then they look at each other, and at Guy, who's trying to keep from smiling, for confirmation. Jake, the older of the younger, is the first to call my bluff.

'Nuh uh! You *do* poo!'

I keep my face completely impassive and shake my head, one eyebrow raised as if I can't believe he didn't know that some people just don't do that. Oscar has spotted a potential chink in my armour: 'Then why do you have a bottom?'

I refuse to be thrown off my guard (or be distracted by my hideous bottom, currently spread across an entire couch cushion). Cool as a cucumber, I reply: 'Because otherwise where would I sit, silly?'

Jake is still unconvinced.

'No! You have to poo! That's why you have a bottom and a bottom-hole.'

'Ah, that's why *you* have a bottom-hole, but mine is purely ornamental.'

I'm not sure at this point that I should continue. After all, isn't discussion of assholes something one should avoid with small children? But I'm having way too much fun to stop now.

'Stop LYING.' Jake is shouting now, but he doesn't rattle me.

'Oh yes, my bottom is there to balance out my shape and to provide comfortable seating, and my bottom-hole is there simply to make me look like everyone else. But it isn't a *working* bottom-hole.'

The boys look like they're caught somewhere between fascination and disbelief. Guy is nodding along with me, trying to add the weight of his older-brother reliability to the argument. For my part, I'm holding firm, giving no indication that what I'm saying might not be true, a trick I learned from my dad.

And speaking of dads, here comes Russell, to check on the fire and generally make sure his newest progeny aren't causing too much trouble for his oldest son's nice American girlfriend.

'Daddy, Daddy!' Jake has fallen back on that last refuge of children: the parental defence. 'Anne says she doesn't poo and her bottom-hole doesn't work.'

Russell turns to me and I try not to laugh. I'm pretty comfortable around him, despite only having met him for the first time a couple of months ago, but this is a whole new line I've crossed. He has a choice to make: either he calls me out in front of his sons or he plays along with what's become a pretty entertaining tease of his youngest children. He turns back to his kids.

'Well, boys, I'm sure Anne would never lie. So if she says she doesn't poo then I guess she doesn't poo.'

Phew. I should have known Russell would be the type to enjoy a little good-natured torture.

The boys stare back at me, in awe. I just raise my eyebrows at them.

'See? Purely ornamental.'

Russell glances at me, a tiny smirk playing on the corners of his mouth, his eyebrows knitted slightly. I can see he's still trying to figure me out. I, on the other hand, have him pegged, and I've decided he's all right.

I give all four boys a smug look, settle back into the sofa, and pull my legs up underneath me. I open my book again and pretend to be absorbed in the words on the page. My stomach grumbles, but luckily it's a quiet one – I cross my arm over my belly and wait for everyone to stop looking at me.

*

Let's get one thing straight before we jump in here: *I don't do that*. By 'that' I mean *poop* and *farts*. Ew. I feel dirty just writing that. Of course it helps to know that they're inevitably someone else's *you-know-what*s I'm referring to, since I don't do that.

I have no trouble at all getting up from a large table of mixed-gender friends and announcing that I have to pee, but when it comes to the *other* kind of bathroom behaviour I'm afraid I just can't go there. Why share such intimate (and icky) things with others? Despite growing up with plenty of hippie cousins and a brother and sister who delight in expelling gas in each other's faces, I've never been comfortable with flatulence or defecation. Which was always fine, even desirable – that is, until I had the surgery.

One of the unfortunate side effects of gastric bypass is that it makes things ... let's say 'finicky' in the belly area. Oh, OK, it makes one *gassy*. Of course, I prefer the term 'airy', not that it conveys the same idea at all. The point is, the section of intestine the doctors bypass is the bit that digests sugars (including lactose) and fats, and when the rest of the intestine, the non-bypassed portion, comes into contact with these substances, it flips out a little. Or a lot, depending on how much funnel cake you've stuffed down it. Ahem.

Anyway, the result is that the intestine throws a bunch of water at the foreign substances, which means that the body gets super-dehydrated, leading to dizziness and faintness, and then of course all the water has to come out somehow ... Suffice it to say, the doctors call this 'dumping syndrome'. And we can just leave it at that, because, again, ew.

I'm pretty good about knowing my limits with fatty foods and sugars, so I've never had this happen in a terribly extreme way. I have been ill, most notably after eating my first and *last ever* real Belgian waffle on a trip to Brussels with Andrea in college, but I'm so controlled (OK, uptight) that it's always been on my terms. There are cruder ways to put it, but let's just say I have a very strong resolve when it comes to politeness (and bottoms). My dad, on the other hand, is not so quick to learn. He's one of the smartest people I know, but he's also seemingly immune to behavioural conditioning. In the experiment where the hamster is offered two cupcakes, one of which is electrified, my dad is the hamster that keeps eating the Red Velvet spark plug.

Most of our celebratory family meals since my dad and I had the GB have ended with him pushing himself away from the table, his main dish half wolfed, his hand clutching his water glass as if drinking a gallon of the stuff could erase his error in judgement. I, on the other hand, have become an expert at pushing around the food on my plate, arranging it artfully until it looks as though I've enjoyed a normal amount, then taking the rest home for lunch the next day.

This isn't to say that I don't have my own issues with the post-GB stomach. Like many post-GB patients, I ended up with a mild-to-moderate case of IBS (Irritable Bowel Syndrome), which basically means that I really *don't* 'do that' often enough, and when I do it's uncomfortable ... that's all the detail I plan on giving, but feel free to Wikipedia it. Also, just because I don't overstuff myself on a regular basis doesn't mean I don't do it occasionally, usually when I'm at a really expensive and delicious restaurant. But my main problem is less to do with lack of self-control and more to do with things outside my control; the worst side effects of the GB, for me, are the gassiness and the effect on my blood sugar.

It doesn't matter where I am or what I'm doing – last time it happened I was on the bus home from work – when a low blood sugar episode hits I'm damn near incapacitated. I get dizzy, my hands shake, and my vision blurs. Sometimes it's so bad I have to sit down, even if that means dropping to the ground on a crowded sidewalk. When it's really strong I get all red and sweaty, and I start panting. My head spins, my heart races, and my limbs twitch. If I'm lucky it happens at home, and Guy can plop me on the couch and bring me a massive glass of water and a square of dark chocolate to try to hasten the end of the episode. If I'm unlucky it happens at a party or an event, and my makeup runs from the sweat and I make a small scene like a swooning Victorian. It's not ideal.

But even the low blood sugar episodes aren't as stressful for me as the windiness. And I don't just mean *farting*, which I prefer to call 'booping', thanks to my family's weird vernacular. Having a bunch of air shifting around in you makes for some interesting noises, even if you're as practised as I am at keeping said air *inside*. That burbling noise you might hear if you sit too close to me isn't burping, it's just a big pocket of air bubbling under my breastbone. And the gurgles and growls that my officemates turn at aren't necessarily related to hunger. Or anything, for that matter. Sometimes it's my fault for chewing gum or drinking coffee on my lunch break, but just as often those noises are the result of nothing at all. Don't mind me, I'm just gurgling over here.

There are times, though, when the bubbles want out. If I'm lucky, I can coax them upwards, in which case I'll just execute a quiet, closed-lipped burp, which I will then subtly blow in the opposite direction of the person I'm with (unless I'm with one of my siblings or Guy has done something cheeky, in which case I blow it in their faces). If it's just Guy and me, in our flat or walking down an empty road, I'll unhook my jaw and let loose, because my inner frat boy needs to be let out sometimes. And if a startled pedestrian rounds a corner and looks at us, wondering where that awful noise came from, I make an appalled face at Guy and give the stranger a *Boys, what can you do?* sort of shrug.

It's possible that my comfort levels have gotten a little out of control in recent years. It's become a source of pride, how loud and shocking my burps can be. But, of course, this is almost always when I'm alone in the flat with my long-suffering boyfriend. Except . . . Well, except when I forget that I'm not alone with Guy. Like the time I was in a restaurant parking lot with my parents and my brother, and I felt at ease, almost as if I *were* in my own flat, and I felt a little pressure in my throat and unthinkingly let it rip. I'll never forget the horror on my mother's face at the monstrous sound that erupted from my open mouth. My brother was too stunned to react at first, and then when he recovered he let out a disgusted 'Jesus Christ, Annie!' I think I saw a twinkle of pride in his eye, though. My dad just *tsk*ed, furrowed his brow, and went back to his BlackBerry.

Since then I've been much more careful about checking my surroundings before belching. Turns out, there *is* such a thing as being too comfortable. But I still maintain I will never, *ever* be comfortable enough, with *anyone*, to boop in front of people.

When I first moved in with Guy, I was worried about the practicalities of this vow. After my freshman year at college, which was spent sharing a room with two other girls, I had managed every year to finagle a single room for myself. So if my belly felt a little bloated or I had a rich meal, I could just go into my room and shut the door for a while (and open the window). But when I graduated and moved to London to live with Guy, that easy privacy disappeared. We shared a tiny, one-bedroom, below-ground flat in Fitzrovia, where sound carried and ventilation wasn't great. Not only that, but Guy was so excited to have me living in his country that he wanted to spend every minute with me. Which was sweet, but, well . . . you know.

I found myself taking advantage of quiet moments in the flat, when Guy was in the living room watching videos on YouTube or reading a Patrick O'Brian novel, to go 'rearrange the bedroom closet' or 'clean the toilet'. I even thought the kitchen, which was more of a hallway between the living room and the bathroom, might be a decent place to relieve some pressure, but I was quickly disabused of that notion one evening. The minute the sound came out of me I froze, one hand on the kitchen table and one over my mouth, afraid to breathe for fear of laughing and giving myself away.

'Honey?' Guy had heard.

I exhaled, slowly. 'Yeah?' Cool and casual. *Boop? What boop?*

'What was that?' I could hear the triumphant grin in his voice, and I was desperate to prove it wrong. I cast about for something that might make a similar noise. I scooched the fruit bowl across the enamel tabletop.

'That?' I crossed my fingers, praying he'd just forget it.

'Um, no . . .' He was almost laughing now.

'Hmm. I don't know.' *It's a mystery!* My heart pounded in my throat – I felt like a trapped sparrow. And then it happened: he started laughing, and he wouldn't stop.

I marched out into the living room, glared at him – his red face, the tears of mirth just forming at the corners of his eyes – and shouted, 'A gentleman would have pretended he didn't hear it!' Then I stormed past him into the bedroom, pausing only to add, 'A *real* gentleman would have taken credit for it!'

That's how weird I am about the lower half of my body – I'd rather get into an argument with my boyfriend than laugh about an accidental bit of gas. For some reason, though, I have it in my head that it's not feminine to have a working digestive system. Oh, it's fine to talk about pee and burp in front of your boyfriend, but God forbid he get wind of anything unpleasant round the back end.

So my own personal GB side effects are difficult – physically, a bit, but mostly in terms of emotional and social discomfort. Still, I'm one of the lucky ones. When we were briefed before the surgery, my dad and I were told about all sorts of less bearable potential problems, from emotional distress (depression, sometimes so bad that the surgery has to be reversed) to physical debilitation (surgical wounds that get infected and don't close up for months, leaving massive scars).

For his part, my dad had already been dealing with the usual gas and 'dumping' issues for a few years when he started getting terrible abdominal pain and was sent in for a further, exploratory surgery to find the cause. They thought it was an intestinal hernia, but they didn't find any evidence, and eventually the pain went away on its own. It was scary, though – a serious reminder of just how traumatic the surgery had been, and how flippant we were, both about deciding to have it and about the relatively mild after-effects we experienced.

Since that little scare, my dad has been fine, with the exception of the odd overly rich meal or attack of low blood sugar. As for those embarrassing noises (and sometimes smells) that emerge from our bodies at inopportune moments, I guess we just have to laugh them off and thank our lucky stars that's all we saddled ourselves with when we paid to have our intestines rearranged.

And my issues with femininity and flatulence? Well, we all tell ourselves a million little lies to get through every day panic attack-free: airplanes just don't crash; that driver will stop for me because I'm in a crosswalk; my partner would never hurt me. What's one more? I can still be pretty and feminine, even if I have a working bottom ... right?

16

St Helena, California, Thanksgiving, 2008

The sky over the Napa Valley is turning a soft shade of pink, with orange streaks where clouds slash it haphazardly. The pool in front of the house is reflecting the colours in a perfect mirror image; it's beautiful, and out here on the deck, alone but for two huge, rented tables set with rented cutlery and plates, it's even serene. I take a breath of chilly air and absorb the quiet for a minute before the goosebumps spring up on my bare arms and I'm forced back inside.

The living room is warm and crowded, and smells delicious, like gravy and meat and rich, hearty vegetables. I'm getting really hungry now; dinner was supposed to start at five, but, as usual, it's 5.20 and everyone is still standing around, drinking wine and chatting and nibbling on the cheeses and nuts set out around the room. I walk past the coffee table, trying to ignore the La Tur and Pecorino that are calling my name and save room for the meal that smells so amazing, and perch myself on the arm of the couch where my cousin is reading a story with her kids. I give her a quick smile and look out at the room, letting the chatter of my family and friends wash over me.

My phone vibrates in my dress pocket and I pull it out and flip it open – it's a new text from Guy, who should be asleep by now. I smile as I read it: COULDN'T GO TO SLEEP AFTER WE SAID GOODNIGHT, SO I READ A BIT AND LAY IN BED THINKING ABOUT YOU. I MISS YOU, BEAUTIFUL, HOPE YOU'RE HAVING FUN WITH YOUR FAM. GOODNIGHT LOVE XX

I can feel myself blushing and smiling, and my cousin pokes my legs and raises her eyebrows.

'What's that about?'

I shake my head. 'Just Guy.'

'Oh, Guy, where is he anyway? He couldn't come this year?'

'No,' I make a sad face, 'he has exams and anyway he couldn't afford to come out for both Thanksgiving and Christmas. I wish he could be here, though – he's never come to Thanksgiving, and I think he'd love it so much. I mean, I know he loves our pumpkin pie because I made it for him last year in London . . .' I try not to think about London, about how much I loved living with Guy in our tiny below-ground flat. My work visa expired after six months, so I quit my job as a receptionist and re-entered the UK from a visit home on a tourist visa, spending my newly free days writing a highly autobiographical first novel. But that visa ran out too, and so did the inheritance money that was paying my rent, so now I'm back in California, loving the sun and the family time and the food but missing Guy and hating going to bed by myself every night.

I guess my cousin can see how I feel, because she gives my leg a little squeeze and says, 'Well, maybe next year.'

I nod and try not to think about it any more. I've found a master's programme in creative writing I want to apply for in London, which would start next fall, and my parents have said they'll support me if I get in, so at least I have somewhat of a plan to get back to my guy. For now, I want to soak up the good parts of being home, not focus on the hole in my heart. *Guy will be here in a couple of weeks*, I reassure myself, *and then you'll have the best of both worlds.*

Catie comes over and flops down on the floor in front of my legs, leaning into me and reaching up to tickle my calves. I shriek and pull them away, then swat the top of her head lightly, mussing her fine blonde hair. She leans her head back and sticks her tongue out at me.

'Did Mom say when we were supposed to start eating?' She makes a face, the one we all make a hundred times during the mad holiday season, the one that says *Does anybody know what's going on?*

'Yeah, well she said five o'clock, but it's already like five thirty. I hope it's soon – I'm not sure how much longer I can resist that cheese!'

Catie laughs and her eyes widen with agreement.

'I know! I haven't eaten all day – I'm saving my Points for seconds on pumpkin pie.' She and Mom have been doing the Weight Watchers thing on and off for a couple of years now, but this is the first time I've lived at home while they're both on. When I first moved back, they'd give it the hard sell every time I complained about feeling fat, but I always declined their exuberant suggestions that I attend a meeting with them. ('You'll *love* the meeting leader, he's so funny!') At first I tried to explain to them that my goal in life is to *not* count calories or subscribe to any sort of system, and rather to work out a lot and try to eat healthily and find some sort of peace with where my body levels out, but after my first two or three explanations fell on deaf ears I gave up. Now I just shoot them warning glares when they're starting to slide into obsessive talk about Points and Jazzercise, or I leave the room if I really can't take it and they won't stop – I think they're starting to get the hint, since they don't invite me to meetings as often as they used to. Now I just roll my eyes at Catie and swallow my usual dismissive comments about how she and Mom don't need to be on diets; I'm trying to be supportive, or at least quiet.

'Yeah, Dad and I went out for lunch earlier, but he wanted to go to that nasty pizza place behind the grocery store in town, and I could barely eat any of my slice because it was so greasy. Of course, he ate half a Philly cheese steak and immediately regretted it.' Catie and I roll our eyes in tandem at Dad's bad habits. I continue, 'Anyway, I'm hungry too. I think we should be able to eat soon, though.'

I look up from her face and try to figure out what's going on in the kitchen, about twenty feet away. My gaze drifts through the dining room, past the long oak table laid with colourful placemats and big, round, stemmed wine glasses, and settles on my mother just beyond, darting around the kitchen island where she's setting up a sort of buffet line of dishes. My father is following her around, talking at her, tormenting her with his constant nattering. Her eyes are widening, her hands coming up to her chest, palms out, as if to push him out of her kitchen, but the wild look on her face just entices him to get even closer. He grabs her around the waist, forcing her to stop what she's doing, which drives her crazy. Her body stiffens and her hands go to his chest to push him off, but he just laughs and grabs her tighter. Finally, she laughs a bit too, a high-strung, desperate laugh, and he lets her go and wanders off to find someone else to torture.

Looks like it'll be me.

'Anna!' His eyes have locked on my idle form and now he's barking at me from the dining room, where he's fiddling with the settings. 'Come help your mother!'

I look past him and see my mom's exasperated face – she shoots me a look that says *Please, just don't provoke him*. But I don't even *want* to irritate my dad (for once); he's already on edge, as he always is at large family gatherings, and somehow in these situations any argument between us is always my fault.

I make a face at Catie, who laughs and steals my seat as I get up and make my way to the kitchen, waving a *Calm down* hand at my dad as I pass through the dining room.

'Hey, Mom, what can I help with?'

'Oh, Anna, fab, if you can put the roods in a bowl with a serving spoon, then it's just a matter of keeping your father's fingers out of the food and getting everybody to come serve him- or herself.'

I scoop the sunset-hued rutabagas – a family tradition, mashed with butter and salt and pepper – into the dish next to the pot and dig through the drawers for a spoon. There isn't a clean one, but there's a dirty ladle in the sink that will do well enough. I wash it and stick it into the pile of mash. I find a spare bit of space on the overcrowded counter and wedge the dish in among the other food – vegetables, mashed potatoes, stuffing, salad, and the just-carved turkey, which is now under attack from my dad's hovering fingers. *He never can stay away for long.* I flick his fingers away from the food.

'Dad, get out of here! You'll be full by the time we say grace.'

'Already am!' He looks pleased with himself, but he's going to hurt later.

'OK, everybody,' my mother's voice rings out and hushes the large crowd in the living room. 'Dinner is served.'

I shrink back out of the kitchen before my dad can order me to serve myself – I hate going first, loading up my plate in front of an audience. Andrew, who is unfortunate enough to have just wandered in with four huge bottles of red wine balanced in his arms, is the next target.

'Ah, perfect, thanks. Now grab a plate – don't let it get cold!' My dad sweeps the bottles out of Andrew's arms and sets to uncorking them right there on the end of the laid table. My mom rushes over to keep him from pushing plates and glasses into one another with his clumsy, aggressive movements.

Andrew lets out an exasperated sigh, but he picks up a plate and starts surveying the food. He goes for the turkey first – an obvious choice – which he slathers with gravy and pairs with a hearty spoonful of mashed potatoes, a mound of stuffing, and a few token vegetables. As he makes his way around the counter, others slowly begin to follow suit. I stand in the dining room, planning my own plate from a safe distance. The roods will make a definite appearance, as they're my favourite Thanksgiving dish, after pumpkin pie. Oh, and Brussels sprouts, of course, the only thing not made by someone in the family; we order them in from a local restaurant, and they're amazing, parboiled then sautéed in butter and cheese and plenty of salt. Next priority is turkey – I'm supposed to be protein-oriented, after all – dark meat, because it's easier for me to digest. Then gravy, just a little drizzle, and a small spoonful of mashed potatoes, just for a taste (I don't even really like them that much, but I always feel like I should, and anyway it's not like I *dislike* them). I'll take some salad too – I'll want it in theory, but because it's not a holiday special it will likely be the last thing I eat, meaning much of it will be left on the plate when I push myself away from it in early defeat. And as much as I tell myself I should, I won't be able to resist the stuffing: big chunks of cornbread and onion, greasy and flavourful from the fat it's absorbed from the turkey. I could eat it by the fistful, if only that didn't mean spending the evening throwing up; just because it's been seven years since the surgery and my stomach is completely healed doesn't mean eating too much of a danger food like carbs won't still block me up.

When the crowd thins, I make my way through the offerings. I arrange my dinner just as planned, always trying to take a little bit less than I want, and knowing that despite this precaution I'll still end up with a half-full plate while everyone else goes back for seconds. Part of me misses seconds, but another part of me (my aching stomach, mainly) reasons that I still get the same overstuffing-myself experience, it's just a shorter journey from hungry to full. When I finish with the food, I turn to head for my assigned seat at one of the round tables on the chilly deck; each place is marked by a construction-paper turkey with the assigned name on it, courtesy of my cousins' kids and my nephew. My turkey is pink – the girls made it just for me.

As I go to leave the kitchen, I pause and take in the scene. Thirty-plus people, family, friends, and a few stragglers added at the last minute, are seated around three tables – the long formal dining table inside holds most of the older folk, with the eldest family member at the head, and the two outdoor tables are heaving with the middle generation, my siblings and cousins and their kids. Everyone is eating, laughing, and drinking huge glasses of deep red wine. The kids, all under ten, are running from table to table, trying to avoid their parents' sporadic discipline and comparing the gifts that were left at their place settings. It's loud, and overwhelming, and crowded, but the whole place smells like roast turkey and trimmings and everyone seems happy. All day the kitchen has been buzzing with anxious activity, and my dad has shouted at me or my mom at least three times since lunch, and later there will be bickering over who has or hasn't done enough cleaning up or which cousin made his or her sibling cry or who gets the prize for best martyr – in this moment, though, as all the prep and planning comes together in this huge family meal, all I see is love.

My dad brushes past me, in a hurry to open another bottle of wine and refill my mom's glass. He's in a good mood right now, and he squeezes my shoulder and grins at me, a bit manically.

'How you doin', Anna? You get enough food?'

'Yup, too much, probably.'

'Well, here, let me help you with that.' He picks up a piece of my turkey with his fingers, swoops it through a puddle of gravy, and pops it in his mouth. I laugh.

'Do you even *have* a plate, Dad? You're going to have to put something in front of you or people will be uncomfortable.'

'Oh, don't worry about me,' he says, 'I made sure the seating chart put me next to Wind.' He gestures with his chin and my eyes follow the path to my cousin's husband, a tall, muscular young man who eats more than most of us put together. My dad will switch plates with him the minute Wind finishes his last bite, thus ending up with an empty plate in front of himself, as if he's been good and eaten all his veggies, instead of picking all afternoon and filling up on crackers and cheese.

'Ahh, I'm envious. I'm just going to have to put my leftovers in my own little Tupperware and eat them for breakfast tomorrow.' I pat him on the arm and move around him, through the dining room and out onto the deck. As I step into the chill and slide the door closed behind me, my cousin looks up and waves me over to the empty seat next to her, just under the heat lamp. I pick a Brussels sprout off my plate and pop it in my mouth, chewing it carefully as I make my way toward my pink paper turkey.

*

One of my main reasons for having the GB was my desire for normalcy: a normal body, a normal social life, and a normal relationship with food. I didn't want to have to constantly scrutinise what went on my plate or in my mouth, and I certainly didn't want my issues with food and my body to affect my social life – there was nothing worse, in my mind, than going out for dinner with friends and spending the whole time fretting over the options on the menu or how I was going to work off dessert. So I went under the knife in the hope that altering my insides might also change the way I felt about food; if the control over what I could and couldn't eat was taken out of my hands, I reasoned, I wouldn't be able to get so stressed out over it all.

To a great extent, that's been true. Once my body had healed from the trauma of the surgery, I did start to relax a bit about food. I worried more about getting protein in every meal than I did about the calorie count (it's tough to worry about calories when you're trying to eat meat for every lunch and dinner), and after a few very unfortunate brushes with overly rich foods my body began to warn me ahead of time if something was likely to disagree with me – with just a sniff of fish and chips, my stomach turns somersaults. My tastes started to change, whether as a direct result of the surgery or simply as a side effect of growing up, or maybe a combination of the two. I stopped wanting things like fried chicken or mashed potatoes simply because they were available, and started listening instead to what my body (and, sure, my mouth) actually *craved*.

I also started loving vegetables. I never hated them, as such – it was never an option, as two out of the three things on our dinner plates as kids were always green – but I'd never actively sought them out, either. But somewhere between the surgery and leaving school to live on my own, I developed a raging affection for veggies – finally, a food preference I could share with my mother! I'm more than a little obsessed with asparagus, despite the fact that I have the smelly pee gene like whoa; I adore zucchini, especially roasted in the oven with a heavy splash of balsamic vinegar; if someone cuts up a red bell pepper near me I'll smell it and risk losing a finger to snatch a piece of the crunchy sweetness before it can be cooked down into mush. In college, when I was eating mostly in the dorms but had access to a shared kitchen, I would sometimes get such a strong craving for a fresh green vegetable that I would trudge to the nearest supermarket (about a mile) and buy tenderstem broccoli or kale or baby spinach, then I'd come back to the dorms, sauté whatever I'd found in my little nonstick frying pan with olive oil and salt and eat it by itself as a snack. It was heaven.

When I first moved in with Guy, he was a second-year medical student, but he didn't have the luxury of living in a dorm where all his meals were available to him pre-cooked. As a result, he was much more comfortable in the kitchen than I was at that point (my knowledge and skill were pretty much limited to the method described above, whether the dish was meat or vegetable-based), but he mostly cooked pasta and curries. I'd never really eaten much pasta growing up – my mom almost never cooks it because she's not that into carbs – and those first few weeks of 'spag bol' nearly every night made me feel hideous. I'd always loved pasta as a kid, likely because it was kind of a restaurant-only treat, but I was learning the hard way how stodgy it made me feel when I ate too much of it. So I started cooking more, and we started having more meals like the ones I grew up on: a lean meat, a green vegetable, maybe a salad if I could handle an extra dirty dish. But I had to learn something else the hard way: eating fewer carbs and more meat and vegetables is expensive. Poor Guy had never spent so much on food, and it was all my fault – he also really missed his jarred curries, which are horrible for my stomach and which I don't like anyway. These days we eat mostly lean meats and veggies, and I encourage Guy to go out for curries with his mates.

That's not to say I don't like carbs. For the first year or so after the surgery, I had to avoid them pretty strictly because they're quite gluey once you chew them, and they used to stick in my stomach and make me throw up. But once my body healed and I learned to chew more carefully, I started allowing them back in, and now there's little I love more than a slice of real San Francisco sourdough, toasted and slathered with salted butter. I would choose really good bread over potatoes or pasta any day, although that's not to say I don't eat pasta or potatoes – I eat pretty much everything these days (except fish and chips, which made me extremely sick the one time I tried it), I just try to pay attention to how the food is making me feel as I eat it, to avoid any nasty surprises.

I even eat sweets now, possibly more often than most of my friends. They're different sweets from the ones I favoured as a kid – I much prefer spices like cinnamon and more subtle flavours to rich, chocolatey desserts – but they're definitely classed as sugary. In the early years after the surgery I was terrified of sugar; I didn't touch the stuff for months, and when I finally did it was one nibble at a time (literally, I kept the same candy bar in my bedside table for a month, nibbling it down until it was too gross and I had to chuck it). Once I realised that I could have some sugar as long as I was careful, though, I stopped being so afraid and started being sensible. And then I stopped being sensible and started being excited that I could eat a cookie and it wouldn't mean I'd eat three, because my stomach would punish me if I did that. It seemed like I'd finally gotten the normal, balanced relationship with food I'd always wanted!

It wasn't really that simple, though. In recent years, I've had to admit to myself that I've developed a bit of a sugar addiction. Discovering that I could have just one cookie and then moving away from home in short succession meant I felt like it was OK to always have sweets around; I knew I wouldn't binge, so what was the problem? Well, the problem was what Guy and I call my 'turnover rate'. I get full much faster than most people, but I also digest much faster, meaning I don't stay full for long. I don't necessarily get *hungry*, but I get not-full within about thirty minutes of finishing a normal meal (i.e. one that doesn't make me sick). So if I eat one cookie and I'm fine, then twenty minutes later I can have another and be fine then too. And that's dangerous for a post-GB body – the doctors warned us that snacking was the one way we were likely to gain the weight back, which is something I'm always scared of happening, and something I work damn hard at preventing. I'm still pretty naughty when it comes to sugar, but I also keep a close eye on my weight and my size, and most importantly my fitness. If I'm going to eat cookies and chocolate, then I have to work out regularly. And I also have to eat my greens, but luckily that's no problem for me.

There *are* some things I just can't have, or that I have to eat in such teeny amounts it's almost not worth it. The food I miss most is cereal with milk – even the smallest bowl of the least sugary cereal, with non-fat milk, will always make me feel gross at best, and hide in the loo for an hour at worst. It makes breakfasts at cheap hotels or other people's houses practically impossible. I also can't have full-fat lattes or more than a few bites of ice cream, and I always have to ask in restaurants if their mushroom/celeriac/chicken soups are cream-based, which is a definite no-no for me. My dad has the same problems, but he's not as good as I am about making sure to ask, and his tastes haven't changed as much as mine have – he's still not so keen on veggies and the resulting discomfort doesn't seem to have turned him off making poor choices much of the time (although he *has* finally stopped ordering pork at restaurants, which almost always makes him throw up because it's so tough). We have fewer FaDaBoTi meals these days, and when we do go out somewhere unhealthy I spend a long time studying the menu and trying to decide what will give me the best balance of indulgence and not feeling ill – often I can find something to suit my purpose, and as long as I'm careful to ask about sauces and make sure I eat slowly, I'm usually OK. Still, all the caution and questions in the world can't *guarantee* me an incident-free meal.

Similarly, I can't overstuff myself without suffering serious consequences. This doesn't bother me on family holidays like Thanksgiving, because I know there will always be leftovers, and if my brother or sister has a particularly greedy glint in his or her eye then I can just squirrel away a Tupperware-full and hide it in the fridge to go back to the next day. But at fancy meals out, especially the *really* fancy ones, which tend to involve multiple courses (and those extra courses they sneak in, like palate cleansers and petits fours!) and a lot of butter in every dish, I usually have to be extremely careful, and still I've learned to resign myself to a miserable hour or two after the meal is over. It's OK with me – I figure the post-meal discomfort is worth the fantastic food my mouth gets to taste before my stomach rejects it – but recently I've started to wonder whether it's unfair to my dining partner, usually Guy.

One of the passions that Guy and I share in life is great food. We love to go to Borough Market and spend far too much money on fancy cheeses and meaty green olives, but we also love to eat at nice restaurants. If we ever have any disposable income, it goes first on travel and second on expensive meals out. In six years with Guy, I've been to some of the most amazing restaurants of my life, but unfortunately I've also been sick at or after most of them. At Per Se, Thomas Keller's place in New York, I had to go throw up in the bathroom *twice* (lovely loos, although I'm not a fan of the full-length mirrors on the backs of the doors). In Paris, we ate at Le Cinq and I was very cautious and did so well I didn't throw up once, but on the romantic walk back along the Seine I got so ill I wasn't sure I'd make it home (I did, but only just). And last week, Guy and I had lunch at our favourite London restaurant, Ristorante Semplice, and although I was OK for most of the meal, I was struck immediately afterwards with such an intense pain in my stomach that we had to call off our plans to wander around Regent Street and check out the post-Christmas sales; it was straight into a cab instead, and I spent the next hour curled up on the sofa. Guy was, for the first time I can remember, more irritated than sympathetic, and it jolted me out of my self-absorbed state and made me understand that I'm not the only one who suffers when my belly ruins a nice day out.

This doesn't always happen, of course. We have plenty of meals where I'm fine – I just don't eat all my food, or I order much more carefully, or I don't get the cheese plate *and* a double espresso (doh!) – but it is unfortunate how often the memory of a special dinner, often for a very special occasion, is tainted by my physical reaction to the rich food. As much as I had the surgery to avoid a life of annoying food stress at the table, I didn't really consider that it's less awkward to spend dinner with friends fretting about calories than it is to have to get up halfway through the main course and go throw up in the bathroom of your favourite restaurant. And it's not just awkward for me; it makes my companion(s) uncomfortable too.

There are certainly times, usually when I'm at dinner with Guy or really craving Cheerios and milk, when I wish I could switch the GB on and off. It would be wonderful to have this internal control ninety per cent of the time, but still be able to indulge in a fancy dinner on my birthday or cereal at Motel 6 on a road trip. But then, if I had control over whether or not I had control, who's to say I wouldn't just switch it off whenever I felt like eating an entire batch of chocolate-chip cookies, or grabbing a Happy Meal when I walk past the McDonald's at the end of my road on a cold, grey day?

No, I had the surgery because I didn't trust myself to always make the right choices, and I needed the controls taken out of my hands. Of course, I still find ways to ignore my stomach-captain's orders, but most of the time I'm pretty obedient, and when I disobey I am *always* punished for it. And that right there, that sense of authority from something outside (albeit inside) myself, is worth the awkward moments and uncomfortable post-lunch taxi rides. At least, it's worth it to me; we'll see if Guy eventually tires of it and starts eating out with someone else.

17

San Francisco, February 2009

The paper blanket thing won't fit all the way around my hips. It makes a loud, crackling noise as I pull it, trying to meet the two edges over my naked butt. When it rips a bit, I give up and just sit on the examination bed, tucking the gown under my thighs in a last-ditch attempt to conceal my nudity. The paper on the bed crinkles under me, and I try not to move, resting my weight on my feet, which I set on the handle of the drawer on the end of the bed. I perch like that, breathing deeply and trying to control my blood pressure, for ages before the doctor knocks on the door.

'Come in,' I call, but it comes out as a whisper. Good thing he's just coming in anyway, his head down as he studies my chart.

'Anne, hi, I'm Dr S.' He doesn't smile, just glances at me and offers his hand to shake. He's old, in his sixties maybe, but not kindly-looking. His hair is grey, his face lined, but he carries himself like my dad when I've not lived up to his expectations: judgemental, condescending, mean.

I smile at him and take the hand he's holding out. I shake

it firmly, never one to 'shake like a fish', as my mom has always said, her mouth curling up into a sneer at the thought of women who can't shake hands like men. If my firm grasp impresses the doctor, though, he doesn't show it. He pulls up his stool and looks back at my chart.

'So, what are you here for today, Anne?'

'Well, just a checkup, really, I guess.' *Does anybody even* say *checkup any more?* Every time I use the phrase with a doctor he or she seems to look at me as if I'm a child, as if only a child would come to the doctor without a clear reason. 'Birth control. I need a prescription for birth control. I'm on the pill already, but I got that from Planned Parenthood and they said I shouldn't use their services like a real doctor, but then I moved to London so I didn't have time to get a recommendation, and now I'm back for a while so I should really get a primary gynaecologist, even though I'm hoping to move *back* to London again, but I eventually want to end up here and you get really good reviews on Yelp . . .' I take a deep breath to reinflate my lungs.

The doctor cracks his first smile.

'Oh, yes, that review site. You know, my daughter is always checking those things, seeing what people are saying about me. She gets really upset when people give me bad reviews.' He shakes his head, as if other people's opinions of him are the furthest thing from his mind.

'Oh, well,' I force a laugh, 'I didn't see any bad reviews! Anyway, some people are just looking for something to criticise.'

He doesn't respond to my attempt at kindness, just looks at my chart and frowns.

'So, Anne, your blood pressure is a little higher than we like to see ...'

I nod, hoping that my red face and obvious jitters will explain that, but then he says what I was hoping he wouldn't.

'... that's probably because you're overweight.'

And here we go.

I shrug and smile a bit, as if this misunderstanding happens all the time.

'Well, it's usually pretty good, but I did walk here pretty fast from up the hill and you *are* the first male gyno I've ever been to, so I guess I was a little nervous.' I try to laugh, but he just shakes his head and frowns again.

'Hmm.' He doesn't sound convinced at all. He reaches for his gloves, but before he puts them on he looks over his shoulder at me, 'You don't want a female in the room, do you? Because apparently now we have to ask that these days –' he rolls his eyes ' and I guess I can get my receptionist to come in for the exam ...'

'What? Oh, no. That's fine.' I can't think why anyone would come to a male gynaecologist if she needs a female in the room, but I'm nervous all the same. *Maybe I should have a woman here. Did I make the wrong choice?* His brow unfurrows and I feel validated, as if I've given the correct answer.

He orders me to lie back on the bed and put my feet in the stirrups. I hate this part. All I can think about is my naked butt popping out from under the gown; the sound of the paper as I arrange myself on the bed; the sweat between my legs where I've had my thighs pressed together as tightly as possible. I arrange the paper blanket thing over my lower half and stare at the ceiling. I hear his glove snap, then the wheels of his stool as he glides across the linoleum floor and appears between my legs.

'OK, you're going to feel a little pinch here.'

For a few miserable minutes, the room is silent. I try to control my breathing, try not to focus on the cold metal or the slimy fingers, try to relax my muscles to make things easier.

The exam is quick. He stands up and takes off his gloves.

'OK, Anne, you can sit up now.'

I do, carefully, making sure the paper blanket stays over my lap as I swivel around. I feel the paper beneath me tear a little, and I move more slowly. The doctor sits back down, across the room from me now. He looks at my chart again.

'OK, well everything seems fine, Anne.'

'Great.' *Can I go now? Can I just have my birth control and go?*

'But you know, Anne, at 196 pounds your weight is way higher than it should be for your height. Your BMI places you as obese.'

Oh God, here we go.

'Yeah, well I fluctuate by about ten pounds . . .' I try to think of what else to say. *You've got my information on your chart. You know I've had weight-loss surgery, and plastic surgery, so surely you must know I'm aware of my failings.*

'You really need to get your weight down, and I mean more than ten pounds. And you especially need to make sure it doesn't go up any more, because that can affect your fertility and we may need to change your birth control, OK?' He stares up at me sternly. I can feel my face getting hot, my legs sweating. *Don't cry. Don't cry.*

'OK.'

'OK then, Anne, I'll write you up a prescription and you can pick it up at the front desk on the way out. But just make sure when you move back to the UK that they don't give you a birth control with less than thirty micrograms of oestrogen, because anything less won't be enough for a person your size. You can go ahead and get dressed now.'

I nod, force a smile, and he's gone. I leap off the crackly bed and grab my underwear and bra. I put them on, then I lean over, my hands on my knees, and inhale deeply. I slowly pull my dress over my head, and slide my feet into my flip-flops, resisting the urge to throw one at the door and hear the slap echo through the office.

I make it out of the building and onto the cool, dark street before I totally lose it. I pull out my phone and furiously text Guy, barely looking up as men and women in suits and heels weave around me. GOD WHAT A TWAT. HARDLY EVEN LOOKED AT ME, DIDN'T ASK ABOUT MY LIFESTYLE, TOLD ME I WAS OBESE!

I'm shaking. When the text has been sent, I keep my phone in my hand and focus on where I'm walking. Three more blocks and I'll be out of the financial district. Ten more minutes and I'll be home.

The phone rings and I answer it immediately.

'Hey, love, you OK?' Guy sounds worried.

'No! That asshole doctor, I fucking *knew* I shouldn't have gone to a male gyno, but like an idiot I thought I was being a wuss and just needed to suck it up!'

'What happened? He told you to lose weight?' Guy knows me well enough by now to understand why I hate doctors' appointments.

'Yeah, but he didn't even seem to put me into context! He took one look at the number on the scale and he thought he knew everything about me. He didn't ask about my diet – my reduced-calorie, track-every-fucking-bite diet, which I've been on for *fucking two months*, and he didn't ask if I work out, *which I do, a fucking lot*, and he didn't ask me anything about the *fucking surgery for weight loss that I had*, which was right there on his *fucking chart*!'

My voice is wobbling and I can feel the tears coming. I don't want to cry; I'm not sad, I'm *pissed*. But here they come anyway. People are starting to stare – I pick up the pace.

'Oh, honey, you know you don't need to lose weight to be healthy. You're healthy already.' Guy's voice is smooth, soothing, but I'm losing it now and nothing can pull me back.

'*I* fucking know that, and so would he if he'd bothered to ask about my fucking lifestyle! But he didn't! Why are doctors such *lazy fucks*?'

Guy breathes in sharply. I feel a little bit bad about ripping on his planned profession, but I'm not going to sugarcoat it.

'I really hope you're different when you qualify. I hope you'll take the time to actually *investigate* your patients' health, instead of just relying on one stupid number to tell you everything! You promise you'll do that?'

'I promise to try, love, but doctors don't always have time to –'

'Bullshit. I paid this doctor *out of pocket*. This wasn't some free clinic or NHS GP's office where they only have ten minutes and the computer data controls what they can and can't prescribe. This guy is a private doctor, who makes assloads of money to spend half an hour with me and tell me *specifically* what I need to do to be healthier. And does he tell me to eat less red meat or work out more? No, because for all he knows I'm a fucking vegetarian who runs marathons. Does he tell me my body-fat percentage is too high, or my muscle mass too low? No, because he only cares how much I fucking *weigh*.'

I'm panting now, and my face is starting to sweat as I begin the long climb up to the top of the massive hill my parents' house is perched on. The tears stopped soon after they started, but my hands are still shaking with righteous indignation. *Why the hell didn't I say any of this to that stupid doctor?*

'OK, that's fair enough. I suppose private practitioners should really take the time . . .'

'You're damn right they should! God, it just pisses me off so much, how people look at one number, whether it's on the scale or the label in my jeans, and think they know anything about me. Like I'm fucking gorging on McDonald's and sitting on my ass all day watching soap operas, instead of eating sushi whenever I can afford it and climbing this god-damn *mountain* every day on my way back from work!'

A woman turns her head to stare at me as she walks past, downhill, and I smile at her as if I'm not huffing and puffing and swearing my way up to the top.

'Honey, you really shouldn't let this get to you so much. You're a good girl, you eat well and you take care of yourself. Just focus on being healthy and –'

'I *am* focusing on being healthy, but it's not like I can avoid doctors for the rest of my life, Guy! I have to get pre-scriptions, birth control and asthma meds and whatever else. I have to have pelvic exams and pap smears and all that gross shit they make me do every year. God forbid I ever get sick, and have to go more often than that!'

'Oh, hon . . .' Guy has clearly run out of answers.

'Ugh, whatever. I'm almost to the top of the hill now, so I'll probably lose reception in a minute.' I pause and gulp some air – ranting and walking uphill is an exhausting com-bination. I try to soften my voice a bit, too; it's not Guy's fault the doctor was a dick. 'Thanks for letting me vent to you.'

'You know you can vent to me any time, love; I'm here if you need me.'

I smile a little, a real smile for the first time since I walked down to the doctor's office over an hour ago.

'I know, honey. Hey, can you give me like half an hour before you call the house to say goodnight? I really need to write down all this ranty roiling crankiness that's inside me.'

'Sure, love. No worries.'

It's getting late in England, and I know he needs to be in bed soon, but I can't talk about anything else until I get this out of my system and written down in some sort of organised fashion.

'Thanks, love. I'll talk to you soon. Love you.'

'Love you. Bye.'

I crest the hill and turn around to look down at the towering buildings below. *Fucking asshole*, I think one more time, then I turn toward my house and head for my computer.

*

There are very few situations in which I feel like the gastric bypass was a waste. No matter how fat or ugly or snubbed by society I might feel on any given day, I always believe the surgery was worth it – worth the pain and the expense and the side effects – for the health benefits. And then I go to the doctor's office.

I was pretty healthy before the surgery, for a girl of my size. I had asthma, but as far as I know skinny kids get asthma too, and that was pretty much the only thing physically wrong with me; my blood pressure was good, my cholesterol was *great*, and I was just as physically capable as anyone my age (I made damn sure of that). I had the surgery for emotional reasons: I wanted to be seen as a normal person, instead of the 300-pound circus fat lady I felt like. And my parents agreed to let me have the GB because they were afraid my physical state would worsen as I got older and, in all likelihood, heavier. I suspect they were right.

For a morbidly obese seventeen-year-old, I was doing fine, but the weight loss only made things better. I exercised more because it wasn't as difficult or embarrassing, I ate better because it felt good (and because I was developing quite a taste for healthier foods), and it's likely that losing a hundred pounds also warded off potential blood-pressure issues and maybe even diabetes. Since my weight hit its lowest point of 175 pounds, the year after the surgery, the number on the scales has crept up by about twenty, but it's mostly stayed level there, within about a five-to-ten-pound range (my dad has also gained some weight back, maybe even a little bit more than I have, but then he got skinnier than I ever did). And yes, my stomach has stretched and now I can eat a smallish normal-sized portion, so yes, I have to be more disciplined now than I was in the early post-GB years, and I'm *absolutely* afraid of gaining everything back, and of course, despite moments of blissful forgetting, I still feel much of the time like that obese girl I once was – which is exactly why I was on that restricted-calorie diet at the time: because I *felt fat*. But normally, whatever issues I may have with the way I look, I can usually feel secure in the knowledge that my weight is no longer a *health problem*. Until I'm told that it is. By a doctor. Who knows absolutely nothing about me beyond the number on the scales.

I typed a long rant about that gynaecologist the minute I got home – I'd been writing random diary entries and basically expelling my emotions into my computer for years, since college, but recently I had begun to blog about my life, specifically my issues with weight and body image. The site didn't have much of a readership – mostly people just ended up there when they Googled 'Why are my earlobes fat?', which was pretty rare – but writing down my thoughts for a theoretical audience made me feel like I was putting them in better order, and I held out hope that maybe, every now and again, someone would come across the blog and relate to it. I hoped it could even be a resource for young people considering GB; I put my email address in the sidebar and opened myself up to questions. But none came, so it really ended up being more of an online diary than a conversation, which was fine, as I still needed somewhere to organise my feelings.

When I got back from the doctor's, I was barely through the front door before I was typing at my computer – all the bile and venom I felt about the medical profession and the world as a whole spewed out into the blogger template. I explained exactly what had happened at the doctor's office, and then I took off my I Am Not A Fat Complainer hat and let loose. As I typed, I imagined channelling my indignant fury into a tirade at the person who'd actually caused it, instead of spewing my rage online, where it was likely hardly anyone would read it.

Hey, dickwad, I get that you see hundreds of patients a year who refuse to look their weight problems in the face, but given the information you have there on your chart, twat, I'm not sure exactly what it is that makes you think I'm one of them. I've probably looked my stupid fucking weight in the face a thousand times over in the past fifteen years, and nearly ten years ago I did something pretty fucking drastic *about it.*

And then I toned down my venom a little bit, tried to make it just as passionate without being quite so vulgar, and sent it into the relative anonymity of the internet:

I'm *so* sorry that I still weigh too much; believe me, nobody is sorrier than I! I'm doing my best to lose more weight, but that's not even the issue. The issue is that weight, as in *the number on the scale*, has damn near *nothing* to do with health in any way. It doesn't take into account height, bone mass, muscle mass, water weight, or a million other tiny factors that can make that number five pounds bigger or smaller in the course of a day, in my case at least.

I continued like that while I wrote the whole post, my fingers flying over the keys and my thumbs violently banging on the space bar as I transformed my angry, vulgar thoughts into angry, thoughtful sentences.

You know, I'm always thinking about this shit, in case you were worried. I fucking never allow myself a moment's peace from checking my weight, trying to gauge my size, and considering which diets/exercises might change my body a little more. Look, asshole, I beat myself up just fine without your help – I do plenty of shaming myself about my body, so I'm not sure why you think I need you to jump the fuck in and join the shame game. I doubt you think I'm over-confident, as I came here in a knee-length, floaty dress with a cardigan over it and imme-

diately curled into myself as much as humanly possible
when you forced me to strip my armor and put on this
crinkly, too-small paper 'gown'.

When are doctors going to stop using the term 'lose
weight' as a substitute for 'get healthy?' [...] I'm as
heavy as I am for multiple reasons, which include extra
fat, of course, but also the fact that carrying around 300
pounds on my frame literally thickened my already-
dense bones (I was told this by the surgeon who performed my GB), and that I have legs of steel (under the
flub) from climbing Telegraph Hill every day.

I'm not suggesting that doctors need to be more
sensitive, but that they need to be *smarter*. More specific. Target the problem, you lazy fuckers! Stop using
'weight' as a catch-all term for what ails the patient! If
I need to be less fat, tell me I need to cut down on my
body-fat percentage. If I need to eat more vegetables/
fewer carbs/less red meat, or exercise more, or drink
more water, or have a frickin' colonic once a month,
then TELL ME THAT. I am *over* the scapegoating of
pounds (or kilos, or stone, or whatever). Everybody
(and every *body*) is different, and people in the medical
profession should know this better than anyone.

The more I wrote, and the more I let my imagined shouting
match with the doctor take shape, the stronger I felt. Sure,
the argument was imaginary, and sure, the blog post would
go unnoticed, but it felt really good to finally acknowledge

that my weight and the way people reacted to it wasn't always a reflection of *my* bad habits or ignorance – sometimes other people's stupidity or prejudices were brought to light too. I felt fiery, and vindicated, and furious, and excited.

Up until that day, I usually tried not to blog about anything outside myself. I tried to focus on how *I* felt, what *I* could do to feel differently. I didn't like the stereotype of the angry fat chick, blaming the media and skinny bitches for all her problems; anyway it seemed like a lot of effort to not only formulate real analysis and arguments about how society views fat people and/or fat women, specifically, but to also have to defend it against people who would point to my size and say I was just looking for excuses. Analysing society had always seemed like a luxury only thin people had, kind of like the way extreme feminism was only taken seriously when it came from a man.

But this time, I had to go there. I had to articulate my anger and frustration with the way the world looks at women, judging us by our numbers, assuming it knows us because we ate a burger in public one time or took the escalator instead of the stairs at the movies. All the hatred and blame I'd been feeling toward 'society', whatever that means, all the vitriol I'd been keeping to myself or letting out in snarky comments under my breath, I let loose onto the internet. And a few people even responded (although no doctors, unfortunately), sparking a short, eloquent debate. And I felt better.

But it didn't change anything about the way doctors (and others) see me. I'm still a number, a walking 'goal weight'.

I'll never forget the day I went for my free-with-signup personal training session at the Bally Fitness near my college dorm. It was senior year, and Courtney and I had decided we would motivate each other to make good use of our new memberships. We went together to the session; our trainers were both young men, muscular and attractive. We wanted to impress them, or at least I did. They asked us what our goals were, what we hoped to get out of our gym member-ships. Courtney went first.

'I just want to be healthier, tone up a bit, and, you know, lose some weight, of course.' She said it offhandedly, like everyone wants to lose weight. 'Of course,' the two young men nodded, then looked over at me.

'Um, well, I just want to get healthier too. And I want to tighten up my arms.' I demonstrated my slightly fleshy up-per arms, nowhere near the bingo wings they once were but not as firm as they had been a year before, when I was doing weights on a regular basis.

My trainer, the shorter but cuter one, cocked his head like a parakeet. 'No weight-loss goal?' He knitted his brow with confusion.

I held my ground. 'Nope, not really.'

He continued to look concerned, glanced over at his buddy for support. I caved.

'I mean, if I happen to lose weight, I'm not gonna com-plain!' I chuckled, they chuckled, and we moved on. *Phew.*

My entire life, people have looked at me and made

assumptions. 'Diet Coke, you said?' *No, I didn't – I don't drink soda often, so when I do I want the real thing.* 'You sure you want whipped cream on that non-fat mocha?' *Yes, I'm sure, it's the best part of this treat and the only reason I don't have full-fat milk is because it makes me ill.* 'No weight-loss goal?' *Fuck off!*

This constant pressure to defy people's expectations makes life more difficult to live than you'd think. Why not just diet and exercise and get thin, right? Well, besides the fact that losing weight isn't a matter of logic for me (in the first week of my latest calorie-counting and gym routine I *gained weight*), there's the small matter of contradictions: if I freak out about my body and restrict myself, I'm doing what people think I *should* be doing, but if I eat McDonald's and take the elevator I'm doing what people already think I do *all the time.* Which is what got me into this mess in the first place, or so they figure. It's hard to know which option offers more defiance. Sometimes I get angry with myself for wanting so badly to just go unnoticed – I wish I could be more of a fighter, more obviously defiant, more vocal, but I always cower under the fear that anything I say wouldn't be taken seriously, that the grain of salt offered by the way I look would be so strong as to override the point I was trying to make. Instead I wuss out, and wish to be normal, and when that fails I try to be passive-aggressively rebellious.

So I take the schizophrenic route, one leg on either path. I work out like a crazy person at the gym, then order a mocha with whip at the coffee shop around the corner, insubordination mingling with the sweat on my red face. I hike up a mountain in Italy with all my skinny friends, then eat gelato at the top. I order a small Greek salad with more vinegar than oil, then spend the rest of the day lazing about doing nothing. It's confusing, but it's better than the alternatives: being fat and lazy or being obsessed with dieting. And in the end, I suppose it's a decent mimicry of what normal people do, this mystery that naturally skinny people refer to as 'balance'.

It works for me most of the time. I happen to enjoy being active, and I also enjoy healthy food, and I mostly spend my time with people who know me really well, which means I'm usually able to feel like I make the choices I do because that's the way I want to live my life. But every now and then, someone new enters my social circle, and I get all aflutter about what I can and can't eat in front of her and how defensive it sounds when I say I walk a lot. And the worst part is, I still have to see doctors.

Recently, in London, where I currently live, I went to a nurse for a birth-control prescription. The method I use costs about $80 a month in the States, and that's assuming I can even get home often enough to stock up. So I figured, if I'm paying taxes over here, why not get my birth control for free?

The nurse was lovely, and she gave me a prescription, but she also warned me that my BMI tips me into the obese category, and if it gets up past 33 the NHS won't give me my combined-hormone method any more. I laughed humourlessly, and when she looked perplexed I explained about my history: the surgery, the weight fluctuations I don't seem to have any control over, the number of times a doctor has told me to lose weight. Her brows softened and she smiled, a little bit sad, and said:

'You know, I'm not always so sure about the BMI. I think it leaves a lot of things out, like muscle mass and bone density . . .'

I could see her searching in her mind for some kind of comfort, or at least an explanation, but I put my hand up and stopped her.

'It's OK,' I said, 'I get it. The NHS is a by-the-numbers system. It's not personal, and I get that.'

She looked relieved, and shrugged her shoulders, as if to say *Sucks for you, dude.* I was just grateful that she'd even paused to try to understand my position – what really infuriates me is when there's no acknowledgement of what I and others have been through, the obvious unfairness of all of our lives. I want to gather the entire medical community and shake them by the shoulders, shouting, 'Just be straight with us, for God's sake – tell us what we need to do to stay healthy, but also come from a place of understanding that we weren't all given the same lot in life from the start. SEE THE NATURAL INEQUALITIES IN HUMANS!' But instead I write my frustrations down, and pray that one or two doctors will some day stumble across my rants and read them, and maybe think about them, and maybe even change their minds a teeny bit.

I blogged about that visit to the nurse, and I pretty much repeated my earlier frustrations, with fewer swear words and more poor-me's instead. The tone of that post is less furious than the first one, more resigned. Sucks to be me, was the implied message. It sucks that I got fat; that the surgery didn't make me skinny enough; that if I want to stay on my preferred birth control I need to make sure I schedule my next doctor's appointment for a light week; that I can't predict when a week will fit that bill. It sucks that I can't even rely on a crash diet to ensure that I fit the NHS's idea of 'healthy' on one specific, pre-planned day of the year. But what really sucks is that I even have to think about all that, when all I want to worry about is being healthy and fit, and fitting into my clothes and onto bus seats.

Most days I'm resigned: yes, it sucks, but it is what it is and being angry or stressed won't change that. Sometimes I even manage to forget about the number on the scales and what it means to the people outside my small social world. Unless I have a doctor's appointment or I read an article about weight or someone around me talks about losing five pounds – granted, these things make up a large portion of my life outside my flat – I can convince myself that I'm healthy. Hey, I say to myself, you walked three miles in your flip-flops just now, by accident! Go you! Or I order a salad for lunch because I want one, and nobody's watching and assuming I'm only allowed to eat raw vegetables, and I pat myself on the back for making healthy choices out of desire rather than social pressure.

But then I run up against it again. When that three-month prescription ran out and I made the appointment to go back and be weighed for a second time, the panic set in.

This time, it wasn't anger and indignation that got me blogging. It was fear, unexpectedly acknowledged and very real.

It turns out I don't just dislike doctors; I'm terrified of them. And I'm afraid that might never change. After two decades of dreading doctor's appointments because of the necessary weigh-in and inevitable lecture to follow, and after all the diets and workouts and surgeries and pep talks I've put myself through in a feeble attempt to get 'healthy' enough to allow me to relax a bit about my body, I'm still scared of doctors. Because every time I go to see one, I'm weighed, measured, and found to be simultaneously wanting and overabundant. The number on the scales still dictates the doctor's approach with me, and that approach is almost always a lecture, which is often impervious to explanations about my history with weight and body image and my current lifestyle.

The judgement is bad enough in and of itself, but worms its way under my skin is my own reflection of the shame they project; inside, under all my anger and bravado, I'm petrified that they might be right. After all, I have very little idea of what my body is *really* like, so who am I to say they're making unfounded claims about it? Maybe, despite what my logical brain would have me believe, I'm actually not healthy; maybe I'm still obese, just never lost enough weight in the first place, and now I'm living in denial of how fat I truly am? *Multiple doctors in two different countries can't be wrong*, I tell myself in my crueller moments, *they obviously know something you don't.* This attitude makes it much more difficult to follow my self-prescribed 'diet plan' of staying active, eating well, ignoring the scales all but once a month or so, and judging myself by how I feel and whether I fit into my clothes.

The majority of my brain is on my side these days; worrying about my weight gets me nowhere but depressed and, in all likelihood, heavier. The emphasis should be on how I feel and how I feel I look, not what I weigh. But there will always be a part of me that believes the cruel voice echoed by doctors, the one that tells me I'm huge, abnormal, and socially unacceptable and I should focus all my energy on losing at least fifty pounds, as soon as possible. Those two opposing outlooks often struggle for power over my mind, and I sometimes worry I'll lose the plot altogether as a result.

I have two choices: diet obsessively and try to bring my weight down to a number that will allow me to pass under doctors' radar (this is unlikely to last long, even if I can achieve success at first), or avoid doctors and any other situation that involves weigh-ins for the rest of my life. And I don't want to do either of those things. I just want to be normal.

Wasn't that the whole point of having the surgery in the first place?

Epilogue

Calistoga, California, summer 2010

We enter a big room where two bathtubs sit, full of something brown and thick, and Courtney and her nurse-lady branch off to the right. They head into a little cubicle and disappear behind a high, white wall. I hear the sound of a shower being turned on; the rush of water against hard tiles reverberates through the room and echoes in my rib-cage, where my heart is starting to beat frantically. My guide leads me into the other cubicle, on the left side, and the showerhead comes into view. *I wonder if there's any chance I can convince her to let me shower with my robe on.*

No such luck. The lady turns on the shower and nods silently at my hands, which are clutching the seam where the two sides of terry meet in front of my belly button. She turns her back, and I take a deep breath, inhaling the steam from the hot shower, laced with the smells of moss and dirt from the mud baths in the centre of the room. I kick off my sandals and slowly untie the belt of my robe, then grab the lapels and hold them for a second. I look over my shoulder to make sure the woman still has her back to me – she does, and in one lightning-quick movement I drop the towel and duck under the stream of hot water. My hands shaking, my heart racing, I rinse off as quickly as I can and then pick the robe up off the floor, holding it in front of me like a security blanket.

'OK,' I say, and the woman turns back around.

She frowns when she sees the robe, then she smiles at me as if I don't understand, and reaches out for it.

'I'll take that for you.'

I look down at the fluffy white fabric and hug it tighter to me for a second. Then I look back up at her outstretched hand.

'Oh . . . thanks.' I hold it out to her, still blocking her view of my body, but when she takes it away from me the cold air hits my wet skin and I can feel every inch of nakedness on display. Goosebumps spring up, running from my hips down to my ankles, and my nipples are hard under my crossed arms. *Well, at least I got that bikini wax last week . . . and my boobs won't be too saggy, since it's cold as hell in here.*

Courtney and I come out of our little cubicles at the same time. We grin at each other, struggling to keep our eyes above each other's collarbones. Her cheeks are pink, as I imagine mine are, and we laugh a little.

I think we're both grateful when the women gesture to the tubs. I want to dive into the dark opacity that's waiting to cover me up, want it to swallow my body and surround it with a thick layer of mud. But when I put my leg in – as quickly as I can, to minimise the amount of time that my legs are spread apart – I realise this 'mud' is more like peat.

There are sticks in it! I look up at Courtney, who also looks surprised, and we lock eyes. We both pause for a second, legs apart, one foot in the warm, gooey bog and one on the cold, wet tile floor, and then Courtney shrugs and gets in. I follow.

The mud is drier than I expected, and fluffier. Unlike a true liquid, it doesn't immediately part and envelop me. For a terrible moment, my hips spread out over the peat, more liquid than the mud itself, but then I pull some soil aside to make space for them and my hips sink slowly into the tub, the brown mass of sticks and water and dirt oozing back over me at a snail's pace.

Once I've arranged the mud over my lower body, I cross my arms over my breasts and wait to sink in further. The stuff is shifting around me, but it feels like I'm sinking into quicksand. I look over – Courtney has leaned her head back against the pillow and closed her eyes. She looks relaxed, while I feel anything but. *How can she relax with sticks poking her and this weird, moussey dirt splooging into all sorts of inappropriate places?* I lean my head back too, pulling some mud up over my chest and letting my arms fall down at my sides.

When I'm completely submerged, I close my eyes and try to force myself to enjoy the experience. The mud is warm, and heavy. I feel encased, like I used to feel when my brother would bury me in the sand at the beach when we were little. The warmth spreads through my body, starting at the skin level and slowly making its way through layers of fat and muscle until I finally feel it in my bones. My body has gone limp, my fingers floating in a fluffy cloud of sticks and clumps of dirt. I listen to the drip of the showerheads, echoing off the tile walls. My heart has calmed, and I feel it beating, hard but slow, just under my throat. I hear a cough, and open my eyes, suddenly reminded that it's not just me in this room.

The nurse-ladies are sitting in the far corner, one of them reading and the other leaning her head back against the wall with her eyes closed. Courtney's eyes are open – she's staring at the ceiling in a zoned-out sort of way. I whisper in her direction.

'Dude, I didn't know there would be *sticks* in it!'

Courtney turns her head toward me and laughs a little.

'Yeah, me neither. I sort of thought it would be more clay-based.'

'*Clay-based*?' Courtney would know the different types of mud bath – she's travelled all over the world and done all sorts of cosmopolitan spa treatments. This is the closest to a spa I've ever been, and from the outside it looks like a cheap motel.

'Uh, yeah, me too. I mean, I just thought it would be more like *mud*. This is like that MiracleGro shit my mom uses when she plants flowers in pots at the house.'

Courtney laughs.

'It *is* like that! Weird. I kinda like it, though.'

'Yeah, you know, I wasn't digging it – no pun intended – at first, but now that I'm really all up in it . . . I dunno, it's kind of comforting.'

Courtney nods, and closes her eyes again.

I guess it's quiet time again. I close my eyes too.

My fingers find their way through the muck to rest on my hipbone. They run themselves over my scar, wider at the hips than it is across my belly. I feel the smooth, tight bumpiness there, move my hands over the bones beneath, then slide them past the bunches of skin and fat at the curve of my hips, those places where I itch to grab great handfuls of myself and pull them off me. I manage to avoid doing that now – it's difficult, but I'm determined to enjoy this experience and reminding myself of what I hate is not the way to do that. I do, however, let my palms cup the tops of my inner thighs, my wrists turning so I can feel the soft curve there where the last plastic surgery didn't take enough of the excess. I allow myself this one brief moment to consider that disappointment, but then I slip my hands out of the space between my legs and run them up the tops of my thighs, forcing myself to feel the muscles and revel in the firmness there, without dwelling on what they look like.

It's weird to feel my body without being able to see it, and I'm kind of enjoying this process now. My skin is beginning to go all soft and slippery, like it did after our dip in the spring in Africa, and at this similarity my heart squeezes itself and my body relaxes a bit. *But I'm not in Africa*, I remind myself. I open one eye and look over at the nurse-ladies, both of whom now seem to be taking a little catnap. *Still, it's not so bad, really. Those ladies probably see a hundred naked women a year, and most of them are probably older, with sagging skin and droopy boobs even worse than mine. They're probably used to it.*

I move my hand back to the peat, away from my body,

and lie as still as I can. I keep my eyes closed and breathe through my nose, smelling water and soil and salt from my own sweat. I listen to the shower drip and feel weightless, supported, and warm. A little smile curls the corners of my mouth, and I finally relax.

*

So, the journey is over, at least physically. No more surgeries on the horizon, no more massive weight loss planned or expected, no more bodily expectations at all, besides functioning as normal. The emotional journey, on the other hand, is more complicated. It doesn't involve a linear itinerary, with plotted stops and scheduled changes. It goes forward, sideways, and backwards at will, unpredictable as a house cat chasing dust mites. And the end, if one exists, is nowhere in sight.

But that doesn't mean that things aren't getting better. Before the gastric bypass, I would never have gotten naked in front of anyone, including my best friend. I was desperate for a relationship, but in retrospect it's difficult to imagine myself having sex with anyone, or even letting anyone touch me. I completely isolated myself and my body; even having someone put an arm around me for a photo made me stiffen.

After the GB, I was more comfortable being touched, but only on my upper body, or maybe my waist if I was standing up straight. I made small steps toward letting people in: I went skinny-dipping in Croatia in the dead of night with my two best friends; I managed to get naked in front of a man, even let him touch areas I'd formerly protected; I bought a bikini, and sometimes I actually wore it. But I was far from comfortable.

Even now – after three cosmetic procedures, ten years to get used to this new body, and a six-year relationship with someone patient enough to push me when I get tired of trying to accept it – I'm not comfortable in this body of mine. It still feels some days like it's holding me hostage. It still sometimes feels like my enemy, like the only thing in my life that I can't either beat or run away from.

It may seem strange, but I think my body and I understand each other even less than we did before the GB. When I was fat that was all I needed to know: *I'm fat*. It was the reason I'd never kissed a boy, the reason I never went to parties, and the reason I was depressed and miserable. It was the go-to answer for everything that bothered me about my life, down to the times when I felt like my parents favoured my siblings over me: *They love them more because they're easier, they're healthy and popular and thin*. I was a burden, and I blamed my fat.

But losing weight complicated things. I was confused – why weren't boys flocking to me, why weren't the popular kids at my high school inviting me to parties, why did I still feel like an outsider in my own family? Again, I blamed my body. I hadn't lost enough weight. I wasn't truly thin. I thought maybe if I removed the excess skin and fat left over from the weight loss, maybe *that* would be my dramatic change.

Still, though, the world went on as usual. Sure, I got a little more interest from boys, but I think that probably had more to do with my confidence levels than anything else. The kind of guys who wouldn't have looked twice at me when I had a leftover belly and saggy arms are the kind of guys who still think I'm fat now. They're the guys I hold up as experts on days when I'd rather be right than happy. The men who are interested in me as I am now, the ones that ask for my number on the street or flirt with me in coffee shops, those guys probably wouldn't have cared if I still had my excess skin. But it was never really about them.

It wasn't about my family or friends, either. It never was and it still isn't. So what's the difference between my relationship with my body now and my relationship with my body before the GB? It's *me*. It's the desire to change the relationship, instead of changing the body. Not that I'd turn down an offer of a free butt lift (I'm not crazy!), but I can recognise when I've been defeated. Or, to use a better word: wrong.

I've been blaming my body for my problems since I was a kid. I would watch other heavy girls, see them flirting with their boyfriends or laughing with a big group of friends, and I would sear with hatred – at my body for not being good enough, at that other heavy girl for not being unhappy like I was, at her group of friends and her boyfriend for being so much more accepting than the small world that surrounded me. But that has never really been the problem. I have had the most amazing friends, friends who thought I was funny and caring and worth being around, even when I was fat. I have a family that loves me and does its best to show that love, and, eventually, I found the boyfriend I'd spent so long pining after: a handsome, loving, supportive guy who won't let me run away from him, or myself.

I'm not saying that I don't have days where I absolutely loathe my body and think that changing it would change everything, again – it's an easy trap to fall back into. I have whole weeks where all I can think is *If only I had the money for more surgery . . .* or *Just one year of really strict dieting, and maybe I'll get down to a single-digit dress size.* Often being thinner or smaller or firmer seems like the answer to all my problems. But in the last few years I've decided something: that's fucked up.

I'm fucked up. I spend far too much time and energy worrying about my body. Obsessing over it. And changing my body hasn't changed that – if anything it's made it worse. Not only that, but I still feel and act like a fat person seventy per cent of the time (and it's been hard work to get that percentage down from a hundred in the early years after the surgery): I still walk sideways down airplane aisles, like a crab, then spend the whole flight folded in on myself with my legs and arms crossed; I avoid the grates in the sidewalks in New York, certain I'll be the heavy straw that breaks their backs; I still won't sit down on public transport unless there are at least two seats available, for spillover. For all the changes my body has been through, I still treat it the same way I did when it was fat.

So, recently, I've been thinking about working on something else: changing my mind. I don't want to live a half-life, held back by my fear of people seeing my body or, worse, having to face it myself. I want to push myself, to own up to the fact that my body isn't perfect, or even normal, but that doesn't mean I have to waste all my time focusing on its imperfections.

I went for the mud bath with Courtney because it scared me. I knew I'd have to get naked, and I knew there would be strangers there. I knew they'd see my cellulite, my scars, and my ugly relationship with my body. But I went, because I'd always been curious, and we were in Calistoga, sort of the spa capital of California, and we didn't have any other plans for the day. I was tired of waiting to do these things until after I was comfortable with my body. I had to face the reality that I might *never* be entirely comfortable with my body. But I'll be damned if something as stupid as my discomfort is going to keep me from experiencing new things. If my discomfort with creepy men didn't make me flee the souks in Marrakech or the clubs in Milan, then how could something as non-threatening as my own body stop me from trying mud baths or massages?

And I'm not going to stop there. Last year, in New York City, I tried on a dress in the SoHo Anthropologie store, and the zipper got stuck on the way down. I was trapped, in a beautiful, expensive, strapless dress, with my naked breasts hanging out and my sweaty face getting sweatier by the minute. I called Guy in to try to work some sort of magic, but the thing wouldn't budge. He looked at my face, my eyelids twitching as I tried to keep from crying, and raised his eyebrows as if to say 'What now?'

I knew what had to be done, and after a moment's hesitation, I actually did it. I took a second to breathe, called the assistant over, and showed her the problem with the zipper (demurely covering my boobs with my forearm). She baulked for a second, then recovered and called the manager on her radio. And thank *God* for the manager, who was a young, curvy black woman with a sexy short Afro and a brisk but friendly manner. She took one look at me and insisted that this had happened before with this particular dress, then ordered the assistant to get the scissors. I closed my eyes and tried not to cry as the sharp blades sliced loudly through the green grosgrain ribbons that traversed the fabric. And then it was over. The manager put a hand on my arm, stated again that 'it was the dress, *not* you,' and bustled off to put out some other fire.

I put my own clothes on and speed-walked out of the store, Guy trailing painfully slowly behind me, wondering aloud whether I wanted to look at anything else. I glowered at him and hissed, 'No, I want to *get out of here*,' and we did. And I spent all day rehashing that terrible five minutes in my head, remembering the slice of the scissors and the sweat on my upper lip, and reminding myself to be thankful for the wonderful manager who knew exactly what to say.

It was traumatising – I still have flashbacks. But it was also a pretty good story, one I got a lot of mileage out of with my friends for the next few months. And even though I'm still mortified, and may be developing a phobia of zippers – I might have to join the Amish and live a quiet, buttoned-up life in the country – I survived. I'd gotten stuck in a dress in a dressing room and had to be *cut out of it*, which was pretty much my worst shopping nightmare, but I'd survived to tell the tale (many times), and that was the most important thing.

It's not an ending as such, but it's a pretty good start.

Acknowledgements

First, I want to thank all the people who helped make this book a reality: my parents, for their strict grammatical expectations when I was growing up, and for their later support of my educational (and sometimes surgical) pursuits; my teachers, for encouraging my writing while at the same time helping me sharpen it; my course director, Julie Wheelwright, for accepting me into the City University program in which this book originated; my lovely agent, Caroline Hardman, for seeing the potential in my work and for holding my hand through some of my most neurotic 'new author' moments; my editor, Sarah Savitt, who has shaped my book with super-human skill, patience, and grace; and everyone at Faber, Christopher Little and Hardman & Swainson, especially those who read my book in the early stages and said unprompted nice things about it when I sorely needed to hear them. Thank you!

To everyone who has ever encouraged me to push past my insecurities and pursue my love of writing, I owe a great debt of gratitude. Specifically: Dan Harder in San Francisco; Bethany Daniels and Kathleen Finneran at Wash U; Neil McKenna and Sarah Bakewell in London; and so many others at various schools (and sometimes on random train or plane journeys). I am especially thankful for my wonderful critique partners, friends, and cheerleaders: Maria Black, Judy Darby, Livia Gainham, Siobhan McKeown, Caitlin Randall, Jackie Robertson, Kusumanjali Shrikant, and Elaine Williams. And to Natalie Appleton, my book buddy, my friend, and my trusted unpaid editor: I owe much of this book and even more of my sanity to you.

For those who have believed in me, those colleagues and friends and family members who have brushed off my self-deprecating comments (or encouraged me to use them for that greater good – humor), I will be forever thankful. To name just a few: Will Arndt, Brittany Bandy, Nancy Barrett, Emily Bilek, Magda Bojko, Courtney Cooper, Becky Clelland, Laura Esch, Tess Evershed-Martin, Rachel Franklin, Miranda Vaughan Jones, Kristina Jutzi, Cate Kellison, Susann Kellison, Juliet Mushens, Andrea Niles, Andrew Putnam, Donald Putnam, Tessa Teichert-Stein, and anyone else who feels he/she should be listed here. You should.

To all the people who love me (and tell me so, even when they don't think I should need to hear it): thank you. I love you too.